KT-464-404

369 0298235

Action Learning in Healthcare

A practical handbook

HAIRMYRES HOSPITAL
LIBRARY
EAST KILBRIDE

DATE   PRICE
04/11/   £29.99

ACCESS NO   CLASS MARK

WA 540 EDM

Action Learning in Healthcare

A practical handbook

John Edmonstone

Leadership, Management and Organisation Development Consultant

Foreword by

Hazel Mackenzie

Head of Leadership
National Leadership Unit
NHS Education for Scotland

Radcliffe Publishing

London • New York

Radcliffe Publishing Ltd
33–41 Dallington Street
London
EC1V 0BB
United Kingdom

www.radcliffepublishing.com

Electronic catalogue and worldwide online ordering facility.

© 2011 John Edmonstone

John Edmonstone has asserted his right under the Copyright, Designs and Patents Act 1998 to be identified as the author of this work.

All rights reserved. No part of this publication may be reproduced, stored in a retrieval system or transmitted, in any form or by any means, electronic, mechanical, photocopying, recording or otherwise, without the prior permission of the copyright owner.

British Library Cataloguing in Publication Data

A catalogue record for this book is available from the British Library.

ISBN-13: 978 184619 536 5

The paper used for the text pages of this book is FSC® certified. FSC® (The Forest Stewardship Council) is an international network to promote responsible management of the world's forests.

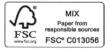

Typeset by Phoenix Photosetting, Chatham, Kent
Printed and bound by TJI Digital, Padstow, Cornwall

Contents

Foreword

John Edmonstone's book is timely. We are living in uncertain times with a great deal of complexity and no easy answers. The tendency towards instant decision-making is swept along by an ever-growing tide of demands on our time. This is the daily reality for many of us both in the workplace and at home. The negative consequences of this 'rush to judgement', as John describes it, are apparent in our histories as individuals, teams, families, organisations and societies.

In this book, John presents action learning not as a simplistic answer but as a means of personal and organisation development which steers a path between action and reflection, and enables the creation of a development culture in our organisations. Action learning moves beyond traditional models of learning, which focus on knowledge and skills, to address the potential gap in terms of transferring that learning into practice.

John sets out the goals of action learning as to:

➤ Benefit organisations by addressing perplexing issues that have previously seemed insoluble
➤ Help organisations to use the potential of their staff better
➤ Help individuals to learn with and from others by discussing the difficulties each member of an action learning set experiences while working on an important organisational issue
➤ Benefit individuals by learning how to survive and operate successfully in a complex and confusing world.

These goals, in themselves, are a testament to the relevance of this book to our current context.

The book is essentially divided into three sections. The first addresses the principles of action learning. It draws on a broad theoretical base including adult learning, organisational development, learning styles, traditional learning and action learning in a way that is simple and accessible, without being simplistic.

The second and largest section of the book concentrates on the practice of action learning. It deals comprehensively with issues including preparing the ground and engaging stakeholders; the scope of action learning; identifying problems, projects and issues; forming and running sets including key skills from the perspectives of set members and facilitator; troubleshooting; managing the process and evaluating action learning. This section of the book is replete with practical guidance and checklists that can be used directly, or adapted. The inclusion of some very helpful chapters on the evolution of action learning and variations on an action learning theme ensures that the content never becomes formulaic but remains thought provoking and invitational.

The final section of the book, combined with the bibliography and web sites, offers a wealth of resources to support action learning and the development of action learning approaches and their applications.

The scope of John's book means that it will have relevance to a broad range of readers including educationalists, managers, those commissioning action learning, OD practitioners, action learning facilitators and set members.

I have known John Edmonstone for close to 20 years. There are few practitioners who can move so deftly between theory and practice in a truly authentic way which resonates and 'makes it real' for those who are fortunate enough to work with him as a commissioner, colleague or as a participant. It is, therefore, no surprise to me that he has created a book which is not a theoretical tome, although it includes plenty of theory, but is truly a user's manual. The book reflects what I have understood as John's compelling drive – to make a difference, not only for the individuals who make up our organisations but also for those who are on the receiving end of our services.

In conclusion and in John's words – 'if what we know about the future is that we do not know much about it, then the key responsibility is not to give people tools that may be out-of-date before they have even been fully mastered, but to help them become more confident and competent designers and makers of their own learning tools as they go along.'

I cannot think of a more pertinent approach to the times in which we work and live.

Hazel Mackenzie
Head of the National Leadership Unit
NHS Scotland
July 2011

Who should read this book?

Potentially, this book has a wide audience. It will be of use to senior managers and professionals considering using action learning for leadership, management and organisation development purposes. It will be of relevance to organisation development (OD) practitioners – those people who have a responsibility for project-managing the use of action learning in local programmes. There is much in the book for the facilitators of action learning sets to take, modify and use in their own practice. Finally, set members themselves will discover material which should enhance their contribution to, and ensure pay-off from, action learning sets.

About the author

John Edmonstone is a leadership, management and organisation development consultant who works in the public sector in the UK. He has held a wide range of line, project and human resource management positions and runs a successful consultancy business based in Ripon, North Yorkshire.

He is Senior Fellow at the School of Public Policy & Professional Practice, University of Keele, Fellow at the Institute for International Health & Development, Queen Margaret University, Edinburgh, Associate at the Centre for Innovation in Health Management, University of Leeds, and Associate at the Edinburgh Institute of Leadership and Management Practice, Edinburgh Napier University.

He has worked regularly with action learning as an internal and external consultant and facilitator since meeting Reg Revans in the 1970s.

Acknowledgements

Thanks are due to all the set members I have worked with over the years in so many healthcare organisations. The insights I have gained from working with you have been immense. Also to all my fellow facilitators, from whom I have learned so much.

Finally, my thanks (as always) to Carol my own personal 'comrade in adversity'.

To
Finlay, Alexander and Madeleine. I know you'll get all the support and challenge you will ever need. May you always stay 'forever young'.

Introduction

I first met Reg Revans, the originator of action learning, at what we would now call a learning disability hospital in the mid-1970s. Although he could some-times come across as the original 'grumpy old man', the clarity and power of his thought and his dedication to action learning as a means of personal and organisational development was abundantly clear. Later, in the 1980s, I recall attending a meeting at the Department of Health in London where Reg tried (and failed) to convince the civil servants running what is now called the Human Resource function that action learning was a method which could help them achieve what they needed – a developmental culture or learning organi-sation within the National Health Service in England.

Subsequent history has involved the use of action learning initially in the development of managers – and then from this base, a spread into other areas – into managerial leadership development; into professional (often clinical) leadership; into professional practice development, and with application to all sorts of professional and occupational groups, including information technol-ogy professionals, risk managers, service-improvement facilitators and so on. Action learning can be argued to have at least some of its' roots in healthcare, based on Revans' pioneering work at Manchester Royal Infirmary in the 1960s[1] and there has subsequently been something of symbiotic relationship between action learning and the UK National Health Service.[2]

History has ultimately proved Reg Revans so right in so many ways. His resignation from Manchester University in protest at the creation of a Busi-ness School on the American model may have seemed 'fogey-ish' at the time (the 1960s), but the insights which he developed then, and afterwards, have recently received a powerful endorsement from no less a figure than Henry Mintzberg.[3]

Of course, action learning can seem deceptively simple and there is a danger of thinking it is only 'learning-by-doing' and that, by extension, anyone can do it, either as a set member or, more particularly, as a facilitator. Revans did not recognise the need for such facilitators, but experience has shown that they are generally now accepted as an integral element of action learning.[4] However, action learning often seems to have developed something of a mixed press in the UK. Among the common instances I have seen when action learning 'goes wrong' are, on the one hand, insufficient challenge offered to set members (and the consequent degeneration of the set into a cosy discussion group); and on the other, fairly prescriptive interpretations and interventions by facilitators (often of a psychodynamic nature). Steering a path between support and challenge as well as between action and reflection remain at the heart of successful sets.

This book is dedicated to the notion that action learning is not that simple and that there has grown up a wealth of experience in its application, so there really should be no need for constantly re-inventing the wheel and repeating the errors of yesteryear. There is, of course, a paradox here. Capturing and sharing such experience helps turn what action learning calls questioning insight (Q) into programmed or codified knowledge (P). Q keeps on developing further insight; therefore, this book can only really be one person's snapshot at one point in time.

The book is divided into three parts. Part 1 is an exploration of the ethos of action learning – the core ideas and underlying assumptions. Part 2 (which is essentially the 'guts' of the book) addresses such issues of practice – preparation, projects, sets, facilitation and evaluation. Part 3 is a compendium of some resources which may be used in association with action learning, together with useful websites and an extensive bibliography. Taken together, Parts 2 and 3 look at the techniques, methods, etc., associated with action learning.

Dotted throughout the book are a number of pertinent aphorisms. It was an approach adopted by Reg Revans himself, as a means of encapsulating complex notions in a simple but effective phrase.

John Edmonstone
July 2011

REFERENCES

1. Revans R. *Standards for morale: cause and effect in hospitals*. Oxford: Oxford University Press; 1964.
2. Brooks C. The role of the NHS in the development of Revans' action learning: correspondence and contradiction in action learning practice and development. *Action Learn Res Pract*. 2010; 7(2): 181–92.
3. Mintzberg H. *Managers not MBAs: a hard look at the soft practice of managing and management development*. Harlow: FT Prentice-Hall; 2004.
4. Pedler M, Burgoyne J, Brooks C. What has action learning learned to become? *Action Learn Res Pract*. 2005; 2(1): 49–68.

Part 1: Principles

CHAPTER 1

What is action learning and what is it for?

'It is impossible for a man to learn what he thinks he already knows.'

Epitectus

There is no shortage of helpful definitions of action learning but at the heart of them all, is the idea that action learning is:

'a method of both individual and organisational development based upon small groups of colleagues meeting over time to tackle real problems or issues in order to get things done – reflecting and learning with and from their experience and from each other as they attempt to change things.'[1]

At first sight this may seem incredibly simple, yet this definition encompasses ideas about both adult learning and organisational change which are both complex and central to what action learning is about.

ADULT LEARNING

Learning is now properly understood as an organismic or natural 'living' process, rather than an ego-driven process.[2] This means that it is not something that 'I' do, but it happens of itself, often in spite of 'I' and not because of it. Learning is also not something confined to formal and structured settings such as primary, secondary and tertiary, education and training events and programmes, but can also be informal in nature – that is, predominantly experiential and non-institutional – and may also be incidental – that is, unintentional and a by-product of other activity.[3]

Derived from the world of adult learning we now know that:

➤ *Learning starts from not knowing*. It is only when people admit that they do not know how to proceed that they become open to learning. There can be no experts in those situations in which there are no 'right' answers and no obvious ways forward. Where there are no such right answers people then must act in order to learn. In that sense action learning involves sharing and exploring our ignorance.

➤ *Learning involves the whole person.* People usually do not, in practice, separate their emotions (or hearts) from their intellect (or minds). The recent popularity of the concept of Emotional Intelligence or EI[4] is a clear recognition of the critical role that emotion plays in both living and learning.

➤ *People learn only when they want to do so*, and not when others want them to do so. Effective learning is therefore self-directed, voluntary, intentional and purposeful. It is an active and learner-driven process rather than a passive and teacher- or trainer-driven one.

➤ A great amount of learning is episodic in nature, rather than continuous. Learning seems to take place in short bursts of relatively intense activity which absorb the learner's attention and is embodied in the phrase 'I'm on a steep learning curve right now!' It typically comes to an end when the immediate purpose of learning has been achieved. People then resort back to a much slower pace of learning before the next such intensive episode takes place, again stimulated by a problem, situation or issue which demands resolution.

➤ *We feel the urge to learn when we are faced with difficulties that we would like to overcome.* These real-world work and life problems provide us with the motivation to learn. We learn best when applying new information or materials to current, real-life challenges and when exchanging feedback with others around these applications. Therefore, people who take responsibility in a situation have the best chance of taking actions that will make a difference. We learn most (and best) when what and how we learn is experienced as relevant.

➤ *Learning is not only about the assimilation of knowledge, but also about the recognition of what is already known.* Learning is inevitably based upon, and builds on, previous experience. It involves both what is taught or read and also our questioning insight. Learning can not only be the acquisition of yesterday's ideas but must also include trying-out new and unfamiliar ideas. It involves asking useful questions in conditions of uncertainty and also involves risk – taking actions that may or may not work.

➤ A powerful block to learning can be a predisposing way of seeing the world or 'mindset' which has been formed by previous experience. These mindsets are made up of our fears, hopes, dreams, speculations, queries, hunches, intuitions, habits, identifications, unconscious projections, half-baked notions, prior training, social conditioning and internalised cultural expectations. They are typically not shared, explicit or even logical when viewed by others, but contribute to the patterns (of beliefs, traditions, fears, conflicts, etc.) that make some things possible and others impossible for each of us. It is our perceptions, values and feelings that tend to get us 'stuck' rather than specific procedures. Everyone, therefore, needs to recognise when their mindset may be no longer be valid, be less useful and in need of review and revision. *People learn best when they are able to question the fundamental assumptions on which their actions are based.* Thus, review and re-assessment of all experience – our knowledge and skills, but also our self-image and personal feelings – is necessary.

➤ Such recognition and revision requires that people have support from others with similar problems and that some of those people come from different settings in order to help stimulate the review process. *Most people are open to learning when receiving helpful and accurate feedback from colleagues who are respected, valued and trusted.* Mutual trust and respect provides strong motivation for learning.

➤ *Learning, and the resulting revision of mindsets, is made easier in a safe and secure atmosphere* – what has been described as a 'holding framework' which can contain people's anxieties with regard to the impact of change and can create the space for them to work on new ways to tackle such issues. Security can be developed by skilful preparation and understanding by a facilitator and from the support of fellow learners.

➤ Learning only becomes possible when someone recognises the need for change and sees the impact of their actions in working on a real problem or issue. *We learn best with and from other people when addressing together pressing difficulties to which no-one knows the solution.* Learning is always for a purpose – clarifying an issue, resolving a problem or living in a more satisfying way. We are motivated to learn when what we learn can immediately be tried out in practice. In action learning, the 'syllabus' is work – the issue, question or problem – and the 'trainer' is replaced by the set members and the facilitator.

➤ Learning is increased when we are asked questions and reflect on what we did; when we are given time and space to address problems; when we can see results; when we are allowed to take risks and when we are encouraged and supported. Learning, therefore, involves cycles of action and reflection. Working on 'out there' problems in the world inevitably leads to learning in relation to personal capacity and emotional involvement. Working on 'in here' issues of personal strengths and weaknesses or likes and dislikes leads to new experiences and growth of capability. The internal world of thoughts and feelings and the external world of action and experience are thus inextricably entwined.[5]

➤ Nonetheless, *the person with the problem is the real expert on the problem.* Unless an individual comes to realise on their own what their problem is, there is little learning to be accomplished by that person.

➤ The role of the facilitator in this process is not to teach, but rather to design, shape and enable conditions from which people can help each other to understand their own past and current personal experience, and the mindsets which derive from it. It is about creating a setting in which learners feel safe and therefore able to review those mindsets, recognise the need for change and see the impact of actions on real problems.[6]

Learners can generally either adopt a deep or a surface approach. In a *surface approach*, the learner is simply trying to gather information one piece at a time and to retain it for the short-term in memory. In a *deep approach*, the learner is intent on understanding an issue and with making connections between experience and new ideas. It is more long-term learning and comes from understanding and internalising something. It is more 'real' in the sense that it is less likely to be forgotten. There is a four-stage process that people pass through with deep learning:

➤ *Unconscious Incompetence*: We do not know that we do not know (or cannot do) something.
➤ *Conscious Incompetence*: We become aware of the fact that we cannot do something or do not know something.
➤ *Conscious Competence*: We have learned it and can do it, often with effort.
➤ *Unconscious Competence*: We can do something 'naturally' and forget that it was ever an issue.

A good example of this is the skill of driving a car. Experienced drivers are at the Unconscious Competence stage, where it feels 'easy' and 'natural', but reflection on the process of starting to learn to drive – the coordination of eyes, hands and feet – recalls how difficult it was originally. As action learning concentrates on what is significant in people's experience, it is essentially an opportunity for deep learning.

A number of practical implications flow from this understanding of adult learning:

➤ Most people do not approach any problem situation in an academic fashion. They are not so much concerned with a subject as with sorting-out their current 'headache'. *People learn best from what they are doing.*
➤ Very few people, therefore, undertake the pursuit of learning in a 'systematic' way – instead, learning is usually limited to the task or problem of the moment. Most people, most of the time, use only those elements of any subject that help them to resolve their immediate problem. *People have an unlimited capacity to learn from experience, but a limited capacity to learn from being taught.*
➤ *Learners do not start with the simple and move to the more difficult – instead, they tackle their problem 'head-on'.* Nevertheless, learners can cope with difficulty and complexity from the outset, provided they can see that they are directly relevant to the learning process.
➤ It is much easier to recognise and adapt your ideas when you have other people around you, facing similar problems, with whom you can talk.
➤ People tend to look for early and practical learning they can apply now, rather than in the future. Thus, there is relatively little interest by most

learners in general principles – few people try to reach general conclusions from specific instances. Once the immediate problem has been resolved, the tendency is to 'store' how to cope with that specific situation, rather than to generate longer-term and more general learning from it. *So learners need help and support (time and structure) to help them to develop their learning beyond the most immediate and particular.*

➤ *Learning also takes time* – so periods of up to twelve months or longer are realistic.

➤ *Individual learning is a visible social process, which may lead to organisational change.*

> 'The word learning denotes change. The word change connotes learning.'
>
> Roger Bacon, 1292

ORGANISATIONAL CHANGE

From the perspective of organisational change and development, it is obvious that the values, assumptions and beliefs underpinning action learning have much in common with the field of Organisation Development (OD). Indeed, there is a case that they are overlapping fields of practice.[7] The continuing major text[8] identifies a number of underlying assumptions about how organisations work:

➤ *The basic building-blocks of an organisation are groups* – so the basic units of change in organisations are groups.

➤ An important change goal is to reduce inappropriate conflict between the different parts of an organisation and the *fostering of more collaborative working within and between organisations.*

➤ Decision-making in successful organisations tends to be located where information sources are, rather than in terms of hierarchical position.

➤ Organisations, parts of organisations and individuals *continuously manage themselves against goals.*

➤ A major goal of a healthy organisation is to develop more open communication, mutual trust and confidence between different functions and professions and between organisational levels.

➤ *People support what they help create* – people affected by a change need to have active participation in the change and a sense of ownership in the planning and conduct of the change.

These values can be summarised as trust and respect for the individual, the legitimacy of feelings, open communication, decentralised decision-making, participation and contribution by all organisation members, collaboration and co-operation, appropriate use of power and authentic interpersonal relations. Taken together, these values, and the practices which flow from them, serve to enhance 'systemic eloquence' – the ability of parts of a system – an organisation, a group of organisations or a network – to talk well to each other.

The most major evaluation of action learning in the Hospital Internal Communications (HIC) programme demonstrated that Action Learning was primarily about organisational change achieved through individual change.[9] A later review of action learning using the Return On Investment (ROI) approach concluded that it had achieved both significant cost-savings and fostered revenue-raising initiatives at an organisational level.[10]

However, in OD terms, action learning is notable for embodying and emphasising an *inside-out process*, based on:

➤ A whole-person focus.

➤ Seeing personal and organisational development as a *'journey, not a destination'* – as operating on the edge of possibility as well as providing people with a map to help them see where they have come from and where they might go.

➤ Seeking to balance support, challenge, action and reflection.

This relates to what has been termed an *intrinsic orientation* to learning, centred on the person and their own learning needs, where the learning is seen to be valuable by the individual in and of itself, and in contrast to an extrinsic orientation, where learning is a means to an end.

In contrast, much of the theory and practice of OD has adopted an *outside-in process* which:

➤ Starts with an emphasis on predetermined or given imperatives and the requirements of specific organisational roles.

➤ From the foregoing produces an 'ideal' state of affairs and models of roles – often expressed in terms of competencies.

➤ Involves processes of appraisal and assessment against the ideal to identify the 'deficit'.

➤ Therefore, sees personal and organisational development as filling the deficit or gap.

This latter approach to organisational change has been called 'instrumentalism' and tends to see action learning as solely as a 'tool' – a means towards reaching previously-defined and wider practical purposes.[11]

> 'The concept of action learning teaches participants to act themselves into a new way of thinking, rather than think themselves into a new way of acting.'
>
> Reg Revans

THE GOALS AND PURPOSES OF ACTION LEARNING

With its' roots in adult learning, and a focus on the inside-out view of organisational change, the goals of action learning are to:

➤ Benefit organisations by addressing perplexing issues that previously seemed insoluble.

➤ Help organisations to ensure that they and their staff reach their fullest potential.

➤ Help individuals to learn with and from others by discussing the difficulties each member of an action learning set experiences while working on an important organisational problem.

➤ Benefit individuals by learning how to survive and operate successfully in a complex and confusing world.

Therefore, action learning has three mutually reinforcing purposes:

➤ To make useful progress on the treatment of a problem, issue or opportunity in real-world terms within an organisation – *to make things happen.*

➤ To help the individual themselves find out how to deal, in future, with other such problems, issues or situations – *to help them to learn how to learn.*

➤ To help those responsible for the development of the organisation (and the people within it) to set in place those activities and support that will help people to create the conditions in which they can learn with and from each other in pursuit of similar tasks – *to help build a learning organisation.*

Action learning appears in different organisations and countries in numerous variants, much as a car is available in many different makes and styles, while still being recognisable as a car!

'Dare to be naïve.'

Buckminster Fuller

Table 1 The Titanic Connection

Reg Revans was the acknowledged 'father' of action learning. An award-winning student of physics at Cambridge University, he also represented Great Britain at the Amsterdam Olympics of 1928. While at Cambridge, working under the supervision of Lord Rutherford, he developed his first original thinking on action learning and experienced first-hand the usefulness of team-working, collaborative thinking and the merits of having views challenged by co-workers.

However, although he was only a small boy at the time, the sinking of the *Titanic* left a lasting legacy in Revans' ideas. His father was the Principal Surveyor of Mercantile Shipping and was deeply involved in the official inquiry into the sinking. The procession of poverty-stricken sailors coming barefoot to his home to report on their experiences aboard the ill-fated liner made a lasting impression on Revans. He heard, time and again, how the sailors had tried to warn those in authority about the risks posed by trying to break the transatlantic record and how these views had been ignored – with disastrous results. The lesson was not lost on Revans. The need to value all views, regardless of hierarchy or status, and the importance of distinguishing between 'cleverness' and 'wisdom' underpinned his ideas on action learning and his advocacy of egalitarian approaches as the basis for learning sets.

'When we focus on changing actions without providing opportunities for individuals to reflect on their values, beliefs and attitudes, we run the risk of building our learning habitat on shifting sands.'

Carl Rogers[12]

REFERENCES

1. Edmonstone J. *The Action Learner's Toolkit.* Aldershot: Gower Publishing; 2003.
2. Claxton G. *Wholly Human: western and eastern visions of the self and its perfection.* London: Routledge & Kegan Paul; 1981.
3. Marsick V, Watkins K. Lessons from informal and incidental learning. In: Burgoyne J, Reynolds M, editors. *Management Learning: integrating perspectives in theory and practice.* London: Sage; 1997.
4. Goleman D. *Emotional Intelligence: why it can matter more than IQ.* New York: Bantam Books; 1996.
5. Beaty L. *Action Learning.* York: Learning & Teaching Support Network CPD Paper 1; 2003.
6. Rogers A. *Teaching Adults.* Buckingham: Open University Press; 1996.
7. Edmonstone J. Action learning and organisation development: overlapping fields of practice. *Action Learn Res Pract.* 2011; 8(2): 93–102.
8. French W, Bell C. *Organisation Development: behavioural science interventions for organisation improvement.* Englewood Cliffs, NJ: Prentice-Hall; 1999.
9. Weiland G, Leigh H, editors. *Changing Hospitals.* London: Tavistock Publications; 1971.
10. Wills G, Oliver C. Measuring the return on investment from management action learning. *Manag Dev Rev.* 1996; 9(1): 17–21.
11. Furedi F. *Where Have All the Intellectuals Gone? Confronting Twenty-first Century Philistinism.* London: Continuum Press; 2004.
12. Rogers C, Freberg J. *Freedom to Learn.* 3rd ed. Englewood Cliffs, NJ: Prentice-Hall; 1994.

CHAPTER 2

Action learning and traditional learning

'Knowledge can be communicated, but not wisdom. One can find it, be fortified by it, do wonders through it, but one cannot communicate and reach it.'

Herman Hesse, *Siddartha*

A large part of the attractiveness of action learning is that it provides a creative alternative to the more traditional approaches to learning. The latter is typically marked by what has been termed a *vicious learning sequence*, as shown in Figure 1.

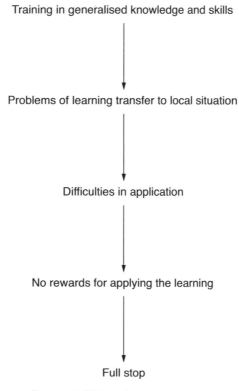

Training in generalised knowledge and skills

Problems of learning transfer to local situation

Difficulties in application

No rewards for applying the learning

Full stop

Figure 1: Vicious learning sequence

Learning which provides learners with generalised knowledge and skills, generally leaves the problem of transferring that learning from the educational institution or training centre to the workplace, almost entirely to the learner themselves. Learners typically experience difficulties in applying learning in their local work situations where there are few rewards (and perhaps even some penalties!) for trying-out something new or different. The result is that action in the workplace tends to come to a full stop. This is often described as the learning transfer problem.

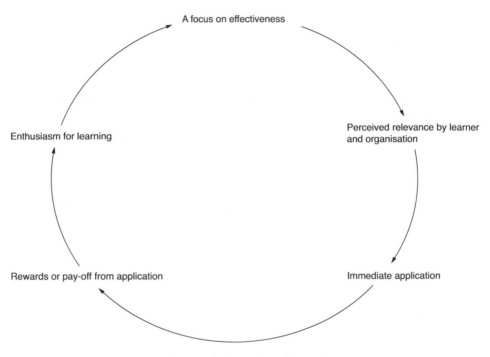

Figure 2: Virtuous learning cycle

Action learning offers instead a ***virtuous learning cycle***, as shown in Figure 2.

In this case, the learning is focused on improving personal and/or organisational effectiveness, with the result that both the learner and the organisation see it as relevant and find it easier to apply. This gives them the learning pay-offs they seek and this success, in turn, increases their enthusiasm for learning in this manner. As Carl Rogers[1] suggested:

> 'Anything that can be taught to another is relatively inconsequential and has little or no significant influence on behaviour. The only learning which significantly influences behaviour is self-discovered, self-appropriated learning.'

Research on learning[2] has identified four distinct modes in terms of the way that learning is used:

➤ *Replicative:* Where learning is prepared and packaged for use in those situations which are marked by the completion of routine and repetitive tasks and which call for little use of any personal discretion.

➤ *Applicative:* Where the emphasis is much more on translating learning into particular prescriptions for action in a range of different situations and occasions.

➤ *Interpretative:* Comprising both understanding, or ways of seeing things from a number of different perspectives, and judgement or practical wisdom made up of an overall sense of purpose, a feel for appropriateness and a flexibility based on a wealth of personal experience.

➤ *Associative:* Learning in a semi-conscious and intuitive way and involving the use of metaphors and images.

Much traditional learning is solely concerned with Replicative and Applicative usage – what action learning calls Programmed Knowledge or 'P' – but action learning potentially covers the entire range, giving as much attention to Interpretive and Associative learning as to the other modes, thus adding Questioning Insight or 'Q' to 'P'.

> 'Tell me, I'll forget.
> Show me, I may remember.
> Involve me and I'll understand.'
>
> Chinese proverb

Michael Polanyi[3] proposed that *'we can know more than we can tell'* and made a useful distinction between explicit and tacit knowledge.

Explicit knowledge is what we can tell. It is knowledge codified into language and therefore communicable to others through documents, instructions, graphs and any medium that can be stored and transmitted. This book is an example of explicit knowledge. *Tacit knowledge*, on the other hand, is personal and context-specific. It is hard to formalise and communicate. It includes the hunches and intuition that tell a doctor that all is not well with a patient and the complex juggling of variables that indicate that something may not be working properly. Polanyi suggests that tacit knowledge tends to be far more extensive than explicit knowledge – the knowledge that can be expressed in words and numbers may be only the tip of the iceberg. Action learning accepts the co-existence of explicit and tacit knowledge. Explicit knowledge is the world of P and there may be a continuous process of making tacit knowledge into explicit knowledge through a series of 'raids on the inarticulate' – of which this book is also, of course, one example.

These ideas are taken further by Nonaka and Takeuchi[4] who see explicit knowledge as what we learn through language or discourse. It is 'book learning' – codified and recorded objective, rational, theoretical knowledge of universal truths, applicable not just in the 'here and now' but also in the 'there and then'. Tacit knowledge they see as what we learn through our involvement with the world. It is subjective, bodily knowledge of the here and now – knowledge by practical acquaintance. It includes our mental models – the paradigms, perspectives and beliefs that guide our actions – as well as our 'action knowledge' – our skills, crafts and know-how. Crucially, it also includes our feelings, hopes, wishes, dreams and ambitions.

Nonaka and Takeuchi, like Revans, stress that these two modes of knowing are partners – they interact with, and change into, each other as we work and learn.

However, a number of common (but false) assumptions unfortunately underlie the more traditional approaches to learning, specifically that:

➤ Learning theory and doing things in practice are quite separate activities.
➤ Theory must be known before practice can be successfully attempted.
➤ Knowing the theory and performing 'routinely' are all that is required.
➤ Learning and improving work practice are merely about repeating routines.
➤ What makes a person expert in their field is their theoretical knowledge.
➤ This theoretical knowledge is itself absolute and unproblematic.
➤ Mastery of theory will ensure mastery of practice.
➤ Theory comes from research and investigation and it is the individual learner's responsibility to apply it unquestioningly to practice.

This leads to an over-concentration of education and training on technical knowledge, and to the creation of a false dichotomy between technical (or explicit) knowledge and practical (tacit) knowledge, as shown in Table 2. It is perhaps not surprising to learn, therefore, that action learning may be difficult to implement in cultures marked by largely didactic approaches to education.[5]

'You cannot teach a man anything: you can only help him find it within himself.'

Galileo

Table 2: Technical and Practical Knowledge (Eraut, 1994)

Technical Knowledge	Practical Knowledge
Typically codified and written	Typically expressed in practice and learned only through experience
Based on established practice	Based on established practice modified by idiosyncratic technique
In accordance with prescription	Loosely, variably, uniquely. In a discretionary way based on personal insight
Used in clearly-defined circumstances	Used in both expected and unexpected circumstances

Technical Knowledge	Practical Knowledge
To meet an envisaged and familiar result	To meet an indefinite or novel result
Emphasis on routine (method, analysis, planning)	Emphasis on non-routine (variety, invention, responsiveness)
Focus on well-defined problems	Focus on poorly-defined problems

This focus on technical knowledge is, of course, exemplified by the popularity of the competency-based approach to education and training. *Competence* is concerned with what individuals know or are able to do, in terms of their knowledge, skills and attitudes. Competency works well with 'tame' issues,[6] where the issue concerned is clear and unambiguous and where tried and tested solutions can be applied. *Capability*, on the other hand, is concerned with the extent to which individual learners can adapt to change, generate new knowledge and continue to improve their performance. Competence suffices when there are high degrees of certainty and agreement, and where the task to be done and the setting in which things take place are both familiar. Capability is required when there is little certainty and agreement, and where both task and setting are unfamiliar. This is the world of 'wicked' issues, where old and unfamiliar solutions do not work, as shown in Figure 3.[7]

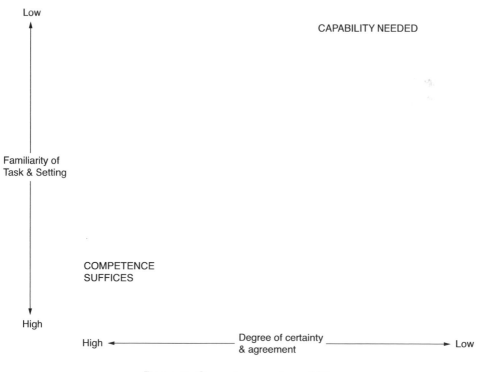

Figure 3: Competence and capability

People have to cope regularly with complex and uncertain situations where previously-operated knowledge and preferred routines fall short or do not fit what is happening. In such cases, what works is not adherence to known and trusted procedures, pretence that surprise elements do not exist, or an expansion of current procedures to 'nail down the problem', but rather:

➤ Reading the situation and responding creatively to what one sees
➤ Drawing on a number of different approaches.
➤ Learning by experiment.
➤ Working by trial and error – systematically.
➤ Turning instinct into insight by thinking about what one is doing as one works and arguing about it in one's head, and with others. This involves theorising about practice during practice.

The challenge in work organisations is, therefore, to develop both competence *and* capability, but the key to survival and success lies more with the latter than the former. Action learning is a creative alternative to more traditional learning. The latter is marked by a prescribed, didactic, expert-based transmission of what worked yesterday, while action learning emphasises relevance, usefulness and a concern with what will work today and tomorrow.

There are also a number of other differences:

➤ Compared with traditional learning, the relationship between theory and practice is reversed in action learning. Theory is created through reflection and dialogue in order to explain and clarify experience, rather than learned (supposedly completely) before experience is attempted.
➤ This results in the lack of any defined 'curriculum' or pre-determined specification of knowledge. This, of course, makes evaluation of action learning difficult because the explicit knowledge to be gained is not specified in advance in any kind of detail, if at all, and may not always be what is originally intended.
➤ Action learning changes the power relationship in the learning situation. Neither the facilitator nor the set member's employing organisation is wholly in charge. Compared with more conventional and formal learning methods, accountability for what is learned remains largely with the individual learner.

> 'What is the sense of knowing things that are useless? They will not prepare us for our unavoidable encounter with the unknown.'
>
> Carlos Casteneda, The Teachings of Don Juan, 1968

REFERENCES

1. Rogers C. *On Becoming a Person*. Boston, MA: Houghton-Mifflin; 1961.
2. Eraut M. *Developing Professional Knowledge and Competence*. London: Falmer Press; 1994.

3. Polanyi M. *The Tacit Dimension*. London: Routledge & Kegan Paul; 1966.
4. Nonaka I, Takeuchi H. *The Knowledge-Creating Company: how Japanese companies create the dynamics of innovation*. Oxford: Oxford University Press; 1995.
5. Pun A. Action learning: encountering chinese culture. In: Jones M, Mann P, editors. *Human Resource Development: international perspectives on development and learning*. West Hartford, CT: Kumarian Press; 1992.
6. Rittell H, Webber M. Dilemmas in a general theory of planning. *Policy Sciences*. 1973; **4**(1): 155–69.
7. Fraser S, Greenhalgh T. Coping with complexity: educating for capability. *BMJ*. 2001; **323**: 799–803.

CHAPTER 3

Action learning: the core ideas

'You must learn by doing the thing. For though you think you know it, you have no certainty until you try.'

Sophocles, 414 BC

L > C

Professor Reg Revans, the originator of action learning, had a scientific background and a liking for expressing some of the core ideas of action learning in the form of mathematical formulae. One such was $L > C$ where L is the rate of individual and organisational learning and C is the rate of individual and organisational change. This implies that both individuals and organisations need to learn faster than the speed at which things change, if they are to have any hope of keeping up. Organisations that continue to embody and express only the ideas of the past are not learning and this is equally true of people. Education and training programmes that teach us to be proficient in yesterday's techniques do not tell us what to do when we meet a new opportunity, but rather make us 'walk backwards into the future'. These ideas seem commonplace in the early years of the 21st century but were much less so when Revans originally formulated them in the 1960s. Later the 1990s produced a flood of ideas and practical methods for developing the learning organisation, many of which derive from Revans's original insights.

'You always got to be prepared, but you never know for what.'

Bob Dylan, Sugar Babe

SINGLE- AND DOUBLE-LOOP LEARNING

The distinction between single- and double-loop learning is most associated with the work of Chris Argyris,[1] although it is also heavily influenced by the work of Gregory Bateson[2] and Donald Schon.[3] Single-loop learning is effectively error detection and correction. It operates like a thermostat on a boiler. If it gets too hot, the thermostat tells the boiler to cool it and the boiler changes its actions to produce a different outcome. People also receive this 'feedback' and where this makes us change our actions (but not necessarily our minds) then this is single-loop learning, as shown in Figure 4. It is the world of every-day, normal and natural 'in-the-box' thinking.

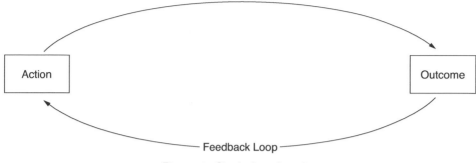
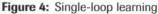

Figure 4: Single-loop learning

In contrast, double-loop learning is where we change our minds about something as a result of the feedback we receive. We may conclude, for example, that a con-tinuing failure to get the outcomes we desire means that we may need to look at our deeper, more fundamental, assumptions with regard to the situation. When a colleague repeatedly rejects our request for help, or when repeated attempts to resolve a problem fail, then we may decide that a deeper enquiry is necessary. We may need to consider, for example, whether we understand the problem situa-tion or in what light we may be seen by that colleague. These 'deeper' questions are typical of action learning and prompt more fundamental change within a system. Double-loop learning (as shown in Figure 5) is less normal and less comfortable because it challenges assumptions, questions 'taken-for-granted' decisions and potentially raises conflict. It represents 'out-of-the box'' thinking.

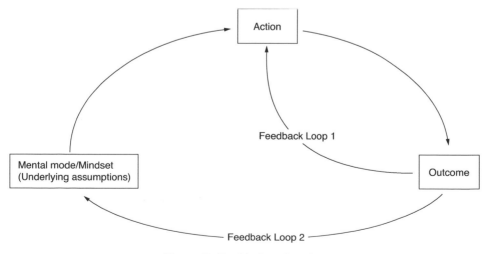

Figure 5: Double-loop learning

Table 3 shows a healthcare example of single- and double-loop learning.

Table 3: Single- and double-loop learning in healthcare

Single-Loop Learning: A hospital examines its' care of obstetrics patients and through a clinical audit, it finds a number of gaps between established standards (derived from evidence-based guidelines) and actual practice. A series of meetings are held in order to discuss the guidelines; changes are then made to working procedures and reporting and feedback on practice are enhanced. The changes increase the number of patients receiving appropriate and timely care.

Double-Loop Learning: In the process of reviewing obstetric care, some patients are interviewed in depth. From this, it emerges that the issues that concern women are to do with convenience of access, quality of information provided, continuity of care and the interpersonal aspects of the patient-professional relationship. As a result of this, obstetric care is radically reconfigured to a system of midwife-led teams in order to give priority to these matters. The standards derived from the evidence-based guidelines are not ignored, but instead are included in a reframed version of values and interactions.

THE LADDER OF INFERENCE

Based upon work by Senge[4] and Argyris[5], this is shown in Figure 6.

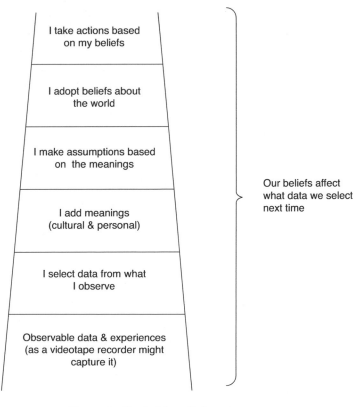

Figure 6: The ladder of inference

Inferring is largely an automatic and unconscious process in adults – we have to operate most of the time using higher-level abstraction, in order to process the huge amounts of information we gather through our senses. Our assumptions or attributions about other people are extrapolations from perceived data at various levels of abstraction – a ladder of inference, where the higher the rung on the ladder, the more abstract and less reliable is the inference.

In the course of our lifetime, our mindsets of attitudes and beliefs become reinforced by our selective attention to events. We tend to pay attention to confirming, rather than disconfirming data. In the main, this is a natural and helpful process because it helps us to avoid information overload and continuous reappraisal of people and situations. However, it does mean that we all operate on the basis of our biases and prejudices – as Simon & Garfunkel sang 'A *man sees what he wants to see and disregards the rest.*' No two people experience the same event in the same way. Thus our natural mental 'shortcuts' – assumptions, expectations, biases, prejudices, beliefs, etc., – can prove to be unhelpful at times.

Problems arise from not testing our attributions about other people's behaviour. The higher the level of inference, the more difficult it is to be explicit about our thinking process and, in threatening situations, it becomes more difficult. Very often, when things 'go wrong' we attribute to others our own weaknesses, assuming that we all fail for the same reasons. We seek to protect ourselves, and others involved, by not telling them the negative attributions we are making about them and this is considered to be the 'right' thing to do. Unfortunately, by avoiding confrontation and leaving attributions untested, they can become self-fulfilling prophecies, even if inaccurate. For example, if I assume someone is autocratic and behave to protect myself from her 'autocratic' decisions, such as avoiding discussion of important issues with her, then she is likely to end up acting autocratically because of what she sees as my untrustworthy behaviour!

So, from our experience, we select certain data to which we add meanings based upon our prior personal and cultural experience. These meanings form the basis of the assumptions we make, and the conclusions we draw. These conclusions enable us to adopt beliefs about the world upon which we base our actions. This is a 'self-sealing' process because the beliefs that we adopt, in turn, powerfully affect the data that we select next time. Only by breaking this reinforcement and examining and where necessary, changing the assumptions, meanings and so on, can double-loop learning take place. Action learning provides a means by which this can happen.

L = P + Q

Sometimes known as the Learning Equation, in this formula, L equals Learning, P equals Programmed Knowledge and Q is Questioning Insight.

Learning is seen to be made up of two main elements and the first, *Programmed Knowledge*, is seen as comprising two elements – external and internal. *External programmed knowledge* is pre-packaged information and skill, prepared for learners by experts, and is contained in a number of 'products' such as textbooks, manuals, checklists, algorithms, handouts, lectures, distance/open learning material, etc. These have all been produced to capture what has already been learned, in order to avoid the learner reinventing the wheel. *Internal programmed knowledge* is made up of our individual mindsets derived from our prior experience, as demonstrated in the Ladder of Inference. An example might be that 'Finance people don't have well-developed people skills.'

'We do not see things as they are, we see them as we are.'

Talmud

Questioning Insight is effectively a process of active listening, questioning and reflecting, leading to review and revision of our personal experience at the edge of our understanding. An example might be a realisation that my own behaviour has stimulated actions in others that have locked us all into a difficult situation – an understanding and acceptance that I am part of the problem too. Questioning Insight arises from inquiry or powerful questions about our own experiences. It is most useful where there is a limited degree of understanding around a problem, and where that problem area is rapidly changing. In that sense it is 'frontier learning' – learning at the edge of our understanding. Q does not cumulatively build our knowledge, but rather helps to reorganise our understanding and see it anew. Participants in action learning learn from generating insights, rather than from collecting knowledge and advice.

There are real tensions between P and Q. P, for example, starts and finishes with answers and instructions, while Q explores what P cannot achieve and forces it to change. If P is pushed – it ultimately produces answers that are harmonious and technically complete. Q creates more questions than answers, and ultimately finishes with a new question. A Q 'state-of-mind' recognises the value of P and accepts it as a co-partner in learning. P, however, only recognises other forms of P.

Nevertheless, there is a real danger of setting-up Programmed Knowledge and Questioning Insight as polar opposites, but they are **both** necessary for effective learning. Providing learners with Programmed Knowledge that is irrelevant to the problem that they face can be disastrous, but so can unfocused Questioning Insight – a form of navel contemplation! Both P and Q are required in this learning equation because neither can be useful in and of themselves. According to Socrates:

'Ignorance is the friend of wisdom.'

The wise do not seek wisdom, only the ignorant! One useful way of seeing the relationship between the two is shown in Figure 7.

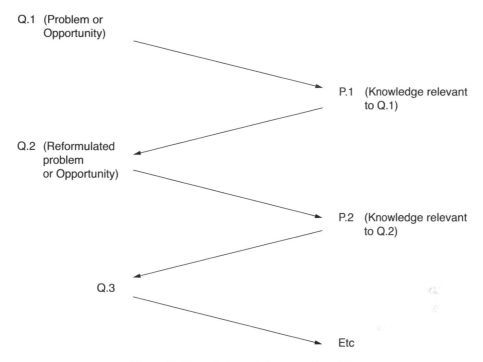

Figure 7: The relationship between P and Q

In Figure 7, a problem (Q1) is explored and it becomes obvious that some Programmed Knowledge (external or internal) is relevant to addressing this problem. After applying this (P1), the original problem is reformulated (Q2). In turn, further Programmed Knowledge (P2) is applied, leading to further clarification of the problem (Q3) and so on. When you begin with Questioning Insight, you often find that some of the existing Programmed Knowledge is of little value, and there may be new Programmed Knowledge that must be acquired or developed. The problem situation does need the application of relevant Programmed Knowledge, but on a 'just-in-time' basis.

Getting the balance right between Programmed Knowledge and Questioning Insight is a major challenge. Too much P and not enough Q can lead to a top-down and didactic delivery of knowledge – therefore, repeating the problems with traditional learning identified in Chapter 2. An over-concentration on Q at the expense of P, means that people may end up 'reflecting on their reflections' and pooling their ignorance without any access to knowledge relevant to their problem situation.

The faster the rate of change that people and organisations experience, the more quickly P becomes out-of-date, therefore, the better our Q becomes (which produces new understanding of the changed situation), and then, the better our chances of personal and organisational survival and growth. This is demonstrated in Figure 8.

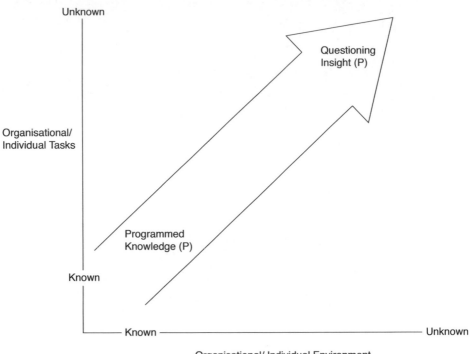

Figure 8: Programmed knowledge, questioning insight and the rate of change

Figure 8 suggests that in those situations where the tasks an individual or organisation has to undertake are well-known, and where the setting in which those tasks take place is familiar, then Programmed Knowledge will largely suffice. However, where both the setting and tasks facing both organisations and people are largely unknown, then there is a corresponding greater need for Questioning Insight. This is the state of affairs facing most people and organisations in the early 21st century.

> 'The unexamined life is not worth living.'
>
> Socrates

BALANCING LEARNING AND TASK CYCLES

Most people recognise the cycle of activity that they follow when they undertake a task, or attempt to resolve a problem. After taking some form of action, there are visible results which are considered, before planning the next action. This is shown in Figure 9.

However, taking action and believing that you have learned from it are not the same as taking action and then reviewing that experience in depth, and with the help of colleagues. A second activity cycle – of learning – is necessary and is shown in Figure 10.

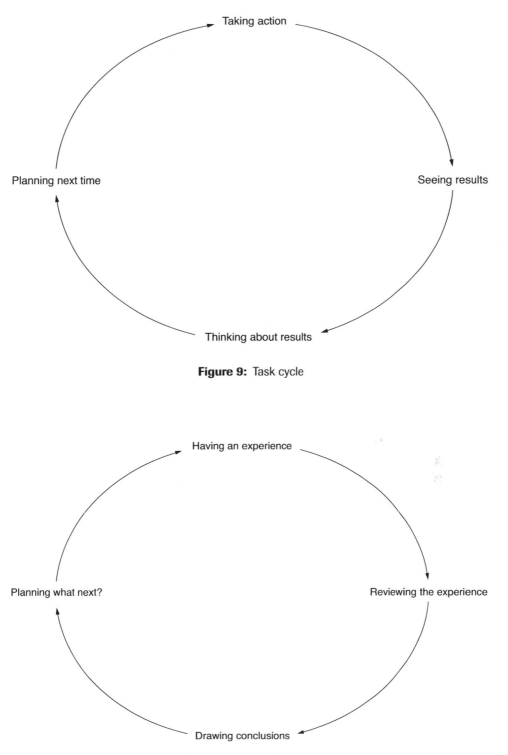

Figure 9: Task cycle

Figure 10: Learning cycle

This activity cycle emphasises the importance of reviewing experience, and concluding what you have learned from it, as the basis for planning what comes next. The reviewing, concluding and thinking about results component of the two cycles are often either forgotten or short-circuited in a culture of both busy-ness and in order to get things done. However, attention to this part of the process is the key to more effective problem-solving and successful individual learning and development.

These ideas were well-expressed by David Kolb[6] who described just such a cyclic learning model, based on two polarities of learning and covering four different learning styles. The first polarity relates to 'concrete experience' versus 'abstract conceptualisation'. Concrete experience involves experience *with* something – an experience that is unique and cannot be transferred in any other way, other than telling someone where to go and what to do, to undergo the same experience. Abstract conceptualisation involves having knowledge *about* something – knowledge which can be expressed in language and, therefore, easily transferred.

The second polarity relates to 'reflective observation' versus 'active experimentation'. Reflective observation involves the internal processing or generation of knowledge by the processes of observing, focusing and reflecting. Active experimentation involves the external processing or generation of knowledge by means of experimenting and acting.

According to Kolb, these two polarities allow four different learning styles:

➤ *Diverging* – where concrete experience and reflective observation are combined. People with a divergent learning style view concrete situations from many perspectives and create relationships between all kinds of aspects and perspectives.

➤ *Assimilating* – where abstract conceptualisation and reflective observation are combined. Assimilators incorporate contrasting observations and reflections into an integrated explanation or theoretical model.

➤ *Converging* – where abstract conceptualisation and active experimentation are combined. People with this learning style combine theory and practice into opportunities for action – devising hypotheses that they can test.

➤ *Accommodating* – where concrete experience and active experimentation are combined. Accommodators achieve practical results by getting to work, trying things out and seeking new experiences.

Kolb reports that most managers and professionals learn and work primarily in the Assimilative, Convergent and Accommodative styles, and that Divergent learning seems to be relatively absent in most professional education – and does not become manifest in most jobs either. A recent evaluation study of action learning[7] concluded that action learning addressed the Divergent learning style more than any other and that Divergent learning was particularly conducive to periods and places of uncertainty, ambiguity and change, when the 'normal' ways of learning do not always apply.

Balancing the task and learning cycles is difficult but can be helped by the idea of 'creative realism',[8] which proposes there is a growing need to devise solutions to problems that are both creative and realistic. However, there seems to be two major tensions in operation. The first is between those approaches to problem-resolution which are practical and realistic in nature, and those which are seen as more idealistic (radical, aspirational). The second tension is between novel (previously untried) approaches and more conservative (based on the status quo) approaches. As Figure 11 shows, this creates four possible options for action.

Conservative Realism: This approach is related to well-established and more traditional ideas. It is very structured and fairly low on imagination and divergent thinking, seeking to avoid any ambiguity and uncertainty. An example would be of an organisation faced with a financial crisis which adopted the knee-jerk reaction of freezing or cutting the training budget.

Creative Idealism: This is associated with 'blue-sky' ideas – original trains of thought which are often fanciful and unrealistic. Faced with the same example as above, a 'single-bullet solution' such as training staff at all levels in the organisation in co-counselling, as a means of personally coping with the crisis, may be implemented.

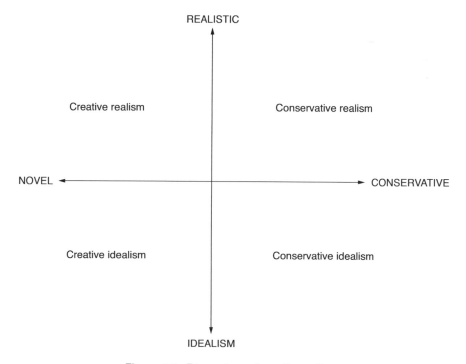

Figure 11: Dimensions of creative action

Conservative Idealism: This involves the extension of common ideas that are unrealistic to begin with – for example, that women are inferior to men at work. These ideas are likely to be unimaginative with little basis in fact, and can often be used to close-down innovative thinking. In the example given, this might involve scapegoating particular minorities (typically on the basis of gender, race, religion, nationality, etc.) as the cause of the financial crisis.

Creative Idealism: Showing imagination and divergent thinking, but grounded in real issues and problems. In the same example, faced with the crisis, a representative grouping of staff may be set up to devise creative routes which see the current financial crisis as providing opportunities, as well as being problematic.

Action learning is concerned with creative realism. It is rooted in the real world but encourages innovative thinking and action to address problems.

INTELLIGENT PERFORMANCE

There is a growing recognition, derived from the development of professionals, that people usually think and do at the same time[9] and that thinking and doing influence each other. We regulate what we do appropriately to the actual situation we find ourselves in – the setting or context that we are in, shapes our reaction. Intelligent performance – where people are thinking about what they are doing as they are doing it – exemplifies a movement to reflecting in practice[10] and does not depend upon previously-learned rules. It is possible to 'do' before the rules are even known, as is demonstrated by small children who can balance on a bicycle without knowing the physics of the activity they are engaged in. We can perform intelligently long before we are able to articulate the principles of our performance. Theory and practice (although separate in some ways) are inter-related and become one in practice. Practice often precedes theory and theorising is a form of practice. Learning to 'do' involves thinking, judgement, decision-making and improvisation. Simply repeating routines is unlikely to improve practice, but more likely to create automatons. To practice successfully involves:

➤ Reflecting on practice.
➤ Drawing-out the theory that underlies our actions.
➤ Relating this to wider theory and practice.

This is just as true of leadership and management as it is for professional practice. Using the metaphor of performing art for the work of managerial leaders it has been suggested of managers that:

> They learn their art by performing it. They discover new depths to the soliloquy, the cadenza, the pas-de-deux, by performing it. Yes, by reflecting on it; yes, by experimenting with it; yes, by repeating it over and over. But all these ways of learning presume that the performers are doing the activities in the first place.[11]

CYCLES OF NON-LEARNING AND LEARNING

It has been suggested[12] that in work organisations (and indeed in life generally) there is what has been called an 'action-fixated non-learning cycle' in operation for most people for most of the time. As Figure 12 shows, people observe a

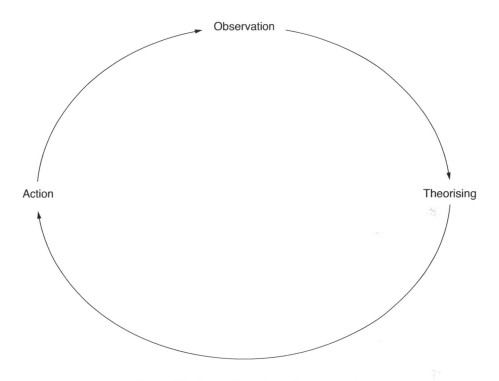

Figure 12: Action-fixated non-learning cycle

problem or situation and in a 'rush to judgement', almost immediately, devise an explanation or theory to explain what is happening, which forms the basis of the action they take to deal with the situation or problem. A more helpful approach is one which interposes the process of reflection at appropriate points, as is shown in Figure 13.

In this action learning cycle there is observation, then a pause for reflection, followed by theorising, and then a further reflective pause before taking action.

This insistence on the need for reflection and review is central to action learning, as is shown in the more enhanced model of what happens in an action learning set. This was developed as part of the Transformational Change Action Learning Project (part of the former NHS National Primary and Care Trust Development Programme) and is shown in Figure 14. Action learning is thus an iterative and experiential process, involving a cyclical notion of learning.

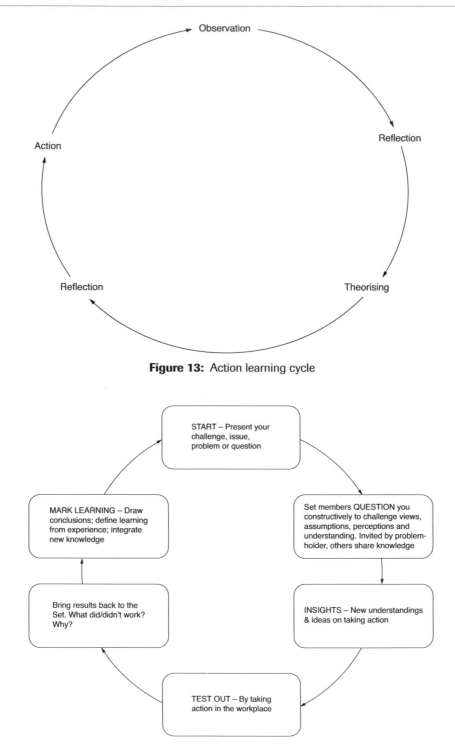

Figure 13: Action learning cycle

Figure 14: Action learning in practice

MINDSETS THAT BLOCK CREATIVITY

Everyone's previous experience helps to form their pre-existing mindsets which can prevent effective exploration of the issue or problem that someone wishes to address. These mindsets could include, for example:

➤ 'There is somewhere a single right answer, if only I could discover it.'
➤ 'It's important to be logical and rational at all times. Imagination is "soft and fluffy" and I'm not that kind of person.'
➤ 'It's important to discover what the "rules" are and to play by them.'
➤ 'At all times you have to decide what's practical – time spent on exploration or dreaming is time wasted.'
➤ 'This is serious stuff. You can't be successful at this and have fun too.'
➤ 'That doesn't fall within my profession/area/remit, so I can't comment.'
➤ 'That sounds fuzzy, unclear and ambiguous – I don't go there.'
➤ 'I need to have an agreed plan before I can go any further.'

The support and challenge that action learning embodies serves to undermine these fixed views of the world and, thus, free-up people for more creative and imaginative work.

COMPONENTS OF ACTION LEARNING

There are a number of key components to action learning. They are:

➤ *Work:* The on-going role or job of a set member, with all the real-time issues, opportunities, experiences which the workplace setting offers.
➤ *Set Member:* An idiosyncratic individual with particular life and work experiences, preferences, styles, etc., who faces workplace and personal challenges and who voluntarily wants to be part of a peer group of people addressing similar issues. Each set member brings to the set their *context* (their unique and personal work setting), their *characteristics* – their personal styles, attributes and preferences and their *challenge* – the work-based issue or problem.
➤ *Sponsor:* A senior manager or professional who has some ownership of the problem and who has agreed with the set member that there are organisational and personal benefits to be gained from participation in the life of the set; who has discussed and agreed the issue or problem with the set member; who gives priority to the set member's regular attendance at set meetings and who provides on-going support and challenge in the workplace throughout the duration of the set and beyond.
➤ *Problem:* The particular 'presenting' or 'starting' issue, challenge or question that the set member has agreed with the sponsor in their organisation at the outset, and that the set member wants to work on in set meetings and back in the workplace. This problem will not only be salient to the individual set member but, hopefully, also to their

organisation and to the other set members. The problem may deal with strategic issues (what to do) or tactical/operational issues (how to do it) and may evolve and change as the work of the set progresses.

➤ *Information:* Knowledge acquired by set members and generated by individual search and research and from interacting with fellow set members.

➤ *Set:* The small and stable group of colleagues voluntarily formed together in a supportive but challenging partnership and meeting over a fixed or agreed timescale to help individuals take action on problems or issues for which there is no readily available answer. The group is committed to the idea of learning from their explorations of the problems. The set is a collective space for thinking and working where every set member acts as a consultant, advisor and devil's advocate for every other member of the set.

➤ *Facilitator:* An individual who sets the scene and acts as initiator, role model, catalyst, etc. for the set meetings and who is particularly active in the early days of the set. The primary responsibility is to support the learning process within the set, including demonstrating exemplary listening skills themselves and making sure that all set members are engaged throughout the set meetings. As the set matures the facilitator may take a more 'occasional' role. Some sets may eventually become self-facilitating or may be so from the outset, with facilitation shared between set members. Facilitation is a way of introducing people to their own learning processes.

➤ *Process:* This involves observation of the problem situation or issue; reflection; the forming of explanations and theories and the taking of action. Factual information about the problem is gathered on an on-going basis. Reflection and theorising take place before, during and after set meetings and action takes place back in the workplace.

> 'The great end of life is not knowledge, but action.'
>
> TH Huxley

REFERENCES

1. Argyris C. *Increasing Leadership Effectiveness*. New York, NY: Wiley; 1976.
2. Bateson G. *Steps to an Ecology of Mind*. Chicago, IL: University of Chicago Press; 1972.
3. Schon D. *The Reflective Practitioner: how professionals think in action*. London: Temple Smith; 1983.
4. Senge P, Kleiner A, Roberts C, *et al*. *The Fifth Discipline Fieldbook: strategies and tools for building a learning organisation*. New York, NY: Doubleday; 1994.
5. Argyris C. *Strategy, Change and Defensive Routines*. Boston, MA: Pitman Publishing; 1985.

6. Kolb D. *Experiential Learning.* Englewood Cliffs, NJ: Prentice-Hall; 1984.

7. De Haan E, De Ridder I. Action learning in practice: how do participants learn? *Consult Psychol J Prac Theory.* 2006; **58**(4): 216–31

8. Finke R. Creative realism. In: Smith S, Ward T, Finke R, editors. *The Creative Cognition Approach.* Cambridge, MA: Massachusetts Institute of Technology; 1995.

9. Claxton G. *Hare Brain, Tortoise Mind: why intelligence increases more when you think less.* London: Fourth Estate; 1997.

10. Ghaye T, Lillyman S. *Reflection: principles and practice for healthcare professionals.* Salisbury: Mark Allen Publishing; 2000.

11. Vaill P. *Learning as a Way of Being: strategies for survival in a world of permanent white water.* San Francisco, CA: Jossey-Bass; 1996.

12. Garratt B. *The Learning Organisation.* London: Fontana-Collins; 1987.

Part 2: Practice

CHAPTER 4

Preparing for action learning

'It is what we think we know already that prevents us from learning.'
Claude Bernard

ASSESSING THE CLIMATE AND CULTURE

The setting or context in which action learning takes place will be a significant factor in the degree of success for both individuals and the organisation or organisations concerned. Settings may be more or less conducive to the likelihood of success, so a helpful early step is to assess whether the climate or culture of the organisation(s) concerned is welcoming, or not, to action learning. There are three helpful tools available for doing this. They are the Organisational Fitness Ranking,[1] the Organisational Readiness for Action Learning Questionnaire[1] and the Organisational Learning Styles Inventory.[2]

The Organisational Fitness Ranking provides some useful questions which might be considered by any organisation, or part of an organisation, before starting with action learning. It directs thinking towards whether action learning should be used to consolidate existing areas of strength or to address areas of 'deficit'. It can also usefully identify the different perceptions of various individuals and groups on such matters.

In the second questionnaire 'readiness' is seen as existing when sufficient challenge to the status quo is balanced with an appropriate degree of openness and support. These readiness conditions are often most prevalent early in an organisation's life-cycle because often when organisations mature (become older, larger and more complex) they tend to lose much of this natural learning ability. In this questionnaire, an organisation, or part of an organisation, rates itself against a set of learning organisation criteria and this offers a helpful guide to the likely value of action learning.

The Organisational Learning Styles inventory is based on a model of organisational learning modes or styles. Using the inventory, it is possible to test out the ways in which an organisation as a whole tends to learn and to spot which modes of learning are underused. By weighting and distributing scores across a range of statements, it is possible to highlight a preference for, or an under-use of, five styles – Habits, Memory, Imitation, Experiment and Awareness.

> 'If I continue to believe as I have always believed,
> I will continue to act as I have always acted;
> And if I continue to act as I have always acted,
> I will continue to get what I have always got.'
>
> Marilyn Ferguson

PREPARING THE GROUND

Organisations tend to use action learning when:
➤ They need to tackle difficult problems or deal with a new and challenging situation.
➤ There is a need to develop leaders who can manage change and uncertainty.
➤ Both personal and organisational development is required.
➤ Traditional, course-based training programmes are inappropriate or ineffective.
➤ Jobs, roles and organisations are changing.

Creating an action learning programme requires careful groundwork if it is to have a realistic chance of success and so, careful preparation is crucial to success. Before anything begins in the organisation it is sensible to:
➤ Read some material about action learning in order to get a feel for what goes on there.
➤ Talk to people who have been members of action learning sets or who have acted as facilitators to sets.
➤ Gain some personal experience in action learning, preferably by being a member of an action learning set.

A CONDUCIVE CONTEXT

While it can never be guaranteed that action learning will 'take' in any setting,[3] there is evidence that a number of factors must be in place to ensure the impact extends beyond the set or sets. They are:
➤ The local system takes a strategic approach to the setting-up of the sets and links them to other relevant activities and networks.
➤ Sets are made aware of the wider context within which they are working, including how their organisations work, who and what they need to influence, and how best to do this.
➤ An influential person (a champion or stakeholder) within the wider system takes a close and supportive interest (either by design or adoption) in what sets are doing and helps them, where appropriate, to grapple with issues.
➤ Proper account is taken of national policies and issues.[4]

This involves attention being paid to the initiation and preparation work necessary to foster a 'structure of welcome'.[5] One aspect of this is the identification of champions or stakeholders.

Champions and stakeholders

'Doubt ascending speeds wisdom from above.'

Reg Revans

Often a local 'champion' in the organisation will initiate or trigger the use of action learning. While this might well be a human resource or training and development person it could also be a senior manager or professional who has had a positive learning experience through involvement in an action learning set. Often these champions develop an idea for the use of action learning and then take it for discussion with other key stakeholders in the organisation or across several organisations. The stakeholders are likely to include:

➤ Senior people in the organisation – the Chief Executive and/or Executive Directors.
➤ Middle-level managers or professional staff who carry responsibility for those staff and their work area potentially taking part in an action learning programme, and who have to arrange cover for the set members who attend set meetings, and undertake work between meetings. These people are key 'gatekeepers' and they need to understand what action learning is, how it works and the responsibilities which will fall upon themselves, as well as 'their' set member(s).
➤ Potential action learning set members.
➤ Potential action learning set facilitators.

There are two principal means by which the original idea may be taken forward, either:

➤ Brainstorming the (as yet) unresolved but burning issues which the organisation faces and identifying the most pressing ones.
➤ Prioritising a list of likely areas to address.
➤ Selecting a work-based topic, theme or project which has to be dealt with anyway and about which no-one really knows what to do. It must be challenging and leading-edge in order to offer the learning required.
➤ Developing a draft proposal based on the above to take to the wider stakeholder group.

or:

➤ Enlisting stakeholder support by asking for volunteers to work on the above, using this to model the activity of an action learning set.

Questions which might be addressed at this early stage include:

➤ Will the theme, topic or project involve set members in real and significant change?

➤ Is what is being suggested feasible in terms of the timescale, resources, experience and skills available?

➤ Are the risks of failure high enough to stimulate action, without being too threatening?

➤ Is the issue or topic unknown enough to need imaginative and creative solutions?

➤ Will the problem or question expose set members to different perspectives and ways of working and learning?

➤ Are senior people in the organisation really committed to the success of the programme?

➤ Does the organisation (or organisations) have the power and will to implement changes arising from the action learning process?

If ownership of the programme is to be established successfully and then maintained, the stakeholders will need to be informed, in plain English, about:

➤ The concept of action learning.

➤ What it will mean for them and their service.

➤ The type and length of commitment and support they will need to provide.

Important selling-points to stakeholders are that:

➤ The workplace is the 'classroom' and its' issues are the learning vehicle.

➤ Learning takes place within the context and culture of action learning programme members.

➤ Action learning facilitates the exploration and testing of current mindsets and helps make the implied or understood more explicit. Thus, action learning promotes reflection.

➤ Action learning promotes openness and trust.

➤ Other learning methods can be 'folded' into the action learning process on a 'just-in-time' basis.

Such 'soft' benefits are not the only way of marketing action learning. A 1996 study[6] of more than 300 managers from twelve countries, set out to determine the benefits to individuals and the return on investment for their organisations resulting from the adoption of action learning. Managers reported a wide range of non-financial benefits to their organisations and to programme participants. Equally important, a £10 million investment in action learning across the organisations delivered a £50 million expected return on investment. Other evaluation studies are not specifically finance-oriented and highlight other benefits accruing from action learning programmes.[7,8]

There is also value in spelling-out, in advance, the responsibilities of all concerned in the workings of action learning. The idea of a *learning contract* may be a useful one. The aim should be to avoid a bureaucratic or heavy-handed approach and to emphasise instead a light-touch and minimalist approach. Nonetheless, there is value in setting out for the set member, sponsor and facilitator exactly what they are signing-up to. An example of this is shown below in Table 4:

Table 4: Responsibilities of Stakeholders in an Action Learning Programme

Set Member

To work with the sponsor to identify and agree an appropriate issue which will be worked on in (and between) set meetings, accepting that the issue may evolve or change as the set progresses.

To regularly attend set meetings and to support and challenge fellow set members as they work on their issues and problems.

To listen attentively to others, and to be open and generous with suggestions and constructive ideas.

To follow-up action agreed at the set meeting back in the workplace and report on progress at future set meetings.

To respect confidentiality and differences and be open to learning through action.

To take part in any evaluation activity.

Sponsor

To become as well-informed about the purpose and process of action learning in general and of the work of the set member in particular in order to make informed decisions and choices.

To carefully identify those individuals for whom participation in an action learning set would be a useful development activity, from the point of view of both the individual and the organisation.

To work with the set member to identify appropriate issues which will be worked on in the set, accepting that these may evolve or change as the set develops.

To support the regular attendance of the set member at set meetings by accepting that set activity is a worthwhile use of time and an investment for the future for the individual and the organisation.

To help the set member with the implementation of actions in the workplace that has emerged from set meetings.

To take part in any evaluation activity.

Facilitator

To model appropriate behaviour, such as high-quality listening skills and asking useful questions, for the set membership.

To be active in the early life of the set in order to foster a sense of collective identity and mutual interdependence among set members.

Thereafter, to be timely and appropriate in interventions in the set's life, concentrating largely on the process (how set members and the set as a whole is working) – with the aim of enabling individual and group learning to take place.

To encourage set members to focus on agreed actions.

To take part in any evaluation activity.

The continuing relationship with key stakeholders is vital and, for the duration of the programme, there is real value in regularly updating and informing stakeholders so they feel both informed and included.

'Doubt is an uncomfortable condition, but certainty a ridiculous one.'

Voltaire

TASTER EVENTS

One way of familiarising people with the possibilities of action learning is through 'taster' events where they can be given a flavour of what it entails. Such a workshop could last one day or a half-day and might involve:

➤ A presentation on the basic concepts underlying action learning.

➤ An opportunity to experience some of the dynamics of a set, possibly through the *Slow Motion Questioning Exercise* contained in the Resources section.

➤ A chance to explore a range of options for future development, including:
  – Intra-organisation or intra-profession sets
  – Multi-organisation and/or multi-professional healthcare sets
  – Multi-agency sets
  – Themed sets based around a problem, topic or role.
  – Kick-start sets, where facilitation is provided for a limited number of early meetings.

There is another paradox here, of course. On the one hand, would-be action learning set members and sponsors need to know enough (in P terms), as early as possible, about action learning in order to make informed choices about whether or not to use it, whether to get involved and so on. On the other hand, it is difficult to really understand what is involved in action learning without experiencing it. Therefore, a fine balance between conceptual material and experiential work needs to be struck in any such event.

WHAT ACTION LEARNING IS NOT

There may be a danger of confusing action learning with other development approaches. Although it may share the characteristics of other types of group work, it is a unique process. So action learning is **not**:

➤ *Group Therapy*: Talking is not enough – set members have to make the leap from intention to action. Moreover, there is no aim in an action learning set to 'peel away' layers of personal meaning. The intention is rather to learn from reflection on experience in order to undertake further action. The focus is therefore more pragmatic and the power remains with the set member, rather than the facilitator.

➤ *A Support Group*: Participants will not benefit if the balance of challenge and support is not right and cosy collusion is a potential danger. The emphasis on action planning for each set member – what they will do when they return to the workplace? – placing responsibility clearly with each individual set member.

➤ *A Blame Group*: Attacking others and blaming them for individual and organisational problems is a sterile activity and unlikely to lead to change.

➤ *Coaching or Mentoring*: It is a group process, rather than a one-to-one process.

➤ *A Task Force or Project Group*: The emphasis is as much on learning as on action.

Action learning differs from these approaches because:
➤ Learning is centred round the need to find a real solution to a real problem.
➤ Learning is voluntary and learner-driven.
➤ Individual development is seen as equally as important as finding a way forward with the problem.
➤ It is a highly-visible social process which may lead to further organisational change.
➤ It takes time.

REFERENCES

1. Pedler M. *Action Learning for Managers*. 2nd ed. Aldershot: Gower; 2008.
2. Pedler M, Aspinwall K. *Perfect Plc? The Purpose and Practice of Organisational Learning*. Maidenhead: McGraw-Hill; 1996.
3. Edmonstone J. When action learning doesn't 'take': reflections on the DALEK programme. *Action Learn Res Pract*. 2010; 7(1): 89–97.
4. Pedler M, Attwood M. How can action learning contribute to social capital? *Action Learn Res Pract*. 2011; 8(1): 27–39.
5. Edmonstone J. Action learning and organisation development. In: Pedler M, editor. *Action Learning in Practice*. 4th ed. Aldershot: Gower; 2011.
6. Wills G, Oliver C. Measuring the return on investment from management action learning. *Manag Dev Rev*. 1996; 9(1): 17–21.
7. Collin A, Sturt J. *Report of an Evaluation Study of an Action Learning Project in Hospitals for the Mentally Handicapped, North Derbyshire Health District*. Sheffield: Trent Regional Health Authority, Organisation Development Unit; 1976.
8. Edmonstone J, Davison V. *An Evaluation of Action Learning Sets Run for the Improvement Network (TIN), Trent Strategic Health Authority*. Ripon: MTDS; 2004.
9. Beaty L. *Action Learning*. York: Learning & Teaching Support Network CPD Paper 1; 2003.

CHAPTER 5

Problems, projects, topics and issues

'A problem is an opportunity in work clothes.'

Henry Kaiser

Action learning is about both the development of people and the addressing of problems in work organisations. It has been suggested[1] that there are two major inputs required for the problem-solving process to be successful. They are:

Hard (or technical) inputs – which are about problem resolution, task achievement, efficient resource use, attention to the bottom line and the meeting of deadlines, targets and objectives. These inputs emphasise the need to be logical, rational, quantifying and structuring, and are expressed in challenge, debate and constructive criticism.

Soft (or socio-emotional) inputs – which relate to personal feelings, motivations and drives. They emphasise the importance of relationships and the need for a secure and safe setting and peer support, where personal experience can be reviewed and re-interpreted.

These two inputs are complementary and cannot, and should not, be separated from one another – and in action learning they are not, as Figure 15 shows.

PROBLEMS

Words like problem, project, issue, topic, theme and question are all used (often interchangeably) to characterise the focus of the work of the set member. This loose definition is quite deliberate. Some people, for example, dislike the use of the term 'problem' and prefer to use 'opportunity'. Whatever it is called, it will be the vehicle for action and learning – so it must be demanding, without being overwhelming. It must address an unresolved issue at role, team, department, service, network, professional, inter-professional, organisational or inter-organisational level. Typically, it will be intractable in nature. Address-

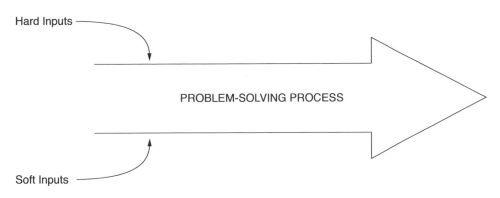

Hard Inputs

PROBLEM-SOLVING PROCESS

Soft Inputs

Figure 15: Inputs to the problem-solving process

ing the problem will not only move the current situation forward, but will also contribute to personal and group learning about how work is done on other problems.

In considering which issues to tackle, it is important that:

➤ The topic to be worked on is *real* and *important to the organisation* and not a contrived exercise.

➤ The challenge chosen is *complex* in nature, dealing with problems which extend across various parts of an organisation or across several organisations.

➤ The problem is *not amenable to an expert solution*, with no ready-made 'right' answers.

PROBLEMS – AND PUZZLES

Action learning makes a distinction between puzzles and problems. With *puzzles*, there is typically broad agreement over what exactly the issue is and some early understanding of what a solution might look like. Although the issue may be complicated, there is an underlying assumption that the facts of the situation can be easily defined, analysed and a single solution found in a sequential manner, not least because previous solutions have been found to this or similar difficulties. There is an existing knowledge-base of tried and tested solutions that it is possible to exploit and we can predict with ease what success will look like. Puzzles have 'best' solutions and 'right' and 'wrong' answers which people have to discover – just like crossword puzzles. They are organisational embarrassments which can be solved by the application of Programmed Knowledge (P) alone (often with the assistance of experts). A puzzle is, for example, the technical process of performing heart surgery – it is complicated, but there is a process for solving it – or writing a business plan for a service within a tightly-structured organisation, especially where the organisation provides staff with highly-specific guidance based on a standardised format and within clearly-defined resource parameters. Other examples of puzzles would be launching a new service or relocating offices. Recent commentators[2] have suggested there is a powerful tendency within healthcare, but not solely confined to that field, to frame what are really problems, as puzzles:

> 'Our learnt instinct … is to troubleshoot and fix things – in essence to break down the ambiguity, resolve any paradox, achieve more certainty and agreement and move into the simple system zone.'[2]

In contrast, ***problems*** are characterised by poor 'focus' and little clear agreement about what exactly the problem is, and by uncertainty and ambiguity about how improvements might be made. The poet John Keats in 1817 coined the term 'negative capability' by which he meant being:

> 'capable of being in uncertainties, mysteries and doubts without any irritable reaching after fact and reason.'[3]

So the concept is not new!

Problems tend to be complex, rather than complicated. They are dynamic rather than static. They sit outside single hierarchies and across systems. They may be novel or they may be recalcitrant – even so intransigent that we have learned to live with them. Childhood obesity is a wicked problem, as is poor communications between health and social care professionals, as evidenced in child protection inquiry after inquiry. Some would even argue that the term 'problem' is a misnomer and that 'enquiry' (embracing messiness and paradox) would be a better replacement, but the word 'problem' will continue to be used here. There is recognition that there are different and valid perspectives, arising from different contexts, cultures, histories, aspirations and allegiances. They are messy, complex, dynamic and interdependent 'tangles' which have no obvious right answers. They are issues which are essentially novel or even unique; where locating the cause(es), explaining and resolving the difficulties, may depend upon the viewpoint of those concerned and where the issue being addressed may well be 'embedded' within another issue. They are things which, if not addressed, will eventually escalate. Problems can be tackled by different individuals in different circumstances and in different ways. At most, resolution might simply mean devising a framework within which all, or most of the stakeholders, could agree a shared definition, devise an agenda for improvement or a process for moving forward – or, at the very least, agree how to live with the mess and make sense of it. Securing the 'right' answer is less important than securing collective consent amongst stakeholders. What is feasible is more important than what is optimal. Success with a problem in one arena is no absolute guarantee of similar success in another arena. While past experience, coupled with Programmed Knowledge (P) can provide a starting-point, simply applying the formula that worked before or elsewhere will probably not lead to success, and may even lead to failure. In this sense, a problem would be providing unlimited health services to all who need them on the basis of limited resources.

The distinction made in action learning between puzzles and problems reflects the similar distinction made between 'tame' and 'wicked' issues.[5]

So the focus of action learning is on problems, not puzzles and these problems should:

➤ *Be real and significant*: The key stakeholders concerned need to care about the issue in question. Failure to address the issue is likely, in time, to provoke a crisis. Ideally, the issue should also be critical and urgent, but experience shows that that there is a tendency for organisations not to entrust such immediate issues to the 'part-time' members of action learning sets and to choose instead issues which are medium to long-term in nature. Whatever issue is chosen, it has to be something which set members can 'get their teeth into' and in which they feel that 'I am part of the problem and the problem is part of me.'

➤ *Involve the set member in action (implementation) as well as diagnosis (analysis):* Set members should be required not only to diagnose and propose ways forward in dealing with issues but also become involved in the often infinitely messier business of putting things into effect. This clearly has implications for the timescale of an action learning programme, as programmes are often time-limited, and this may not always match the realistic timescale for action. Ideally, the issue chosen should lie within the set member's sphere of influence or they should be given the authority to carry matters to a conclusion.

➤ *Be a challenge*: The issue chosen should be something new which the set member has not previously addressed and which they both want and are able to progress. It should be 'hurting' right now and the status quo should not be an option.

➤ *Be defined in some way*: The issues chosen will range along a continuum from tightly-focused to loosely-focused. Tightly-focused issues will be defined in terms of the time and other resources available to address them or in the light of the abilities and learning needs of the set members to address them. An example might be the merging of two departments within a defined time-period. Loosely-focused issues can often be helpful to set members, particularly if they come from a particular professional background with a related mindset which encourages them to see problems in a particular way. The more loosely-focused and open-ended the issue, the more the set member may be inclined to cope with different perspectives and learn to live with a greater degree of ambiguity than before, thus preparing them for future challenges. A loosely-focused issue might be the exploration of a possible new service to service-users. Whatever the style of definition, all set members will need to address such basic questions as 'Whose problem is this?', 'Why is it seen as a problem?' and 'Is the problem, as presented, symptomatic of something deeper?'

➤ *Be capable of being learned from*: Set members should be able to report-back at set meetings on progress (action) and personal insight (learning). The issue chosen should not, therefore, be so specialised or obtuse that the other set members do not feel able to challenge and support the set member in the way they address the problem.

In most cases, set members will bring their own issue, question or problem to the set, but sometimes a set will address a common problem. For example, in a multi-agency set run in Stoke-on-Trent in 2004–05[5] set members collectively addressed 'street-level' issues such as anti-social behaviour and graffiti, which were of acute concern to local communities. In either case, the standard is the same – the issues must be real (unresolved and of considerable significance).

> 'It isn't that they can't see the solution,
> It is that they can't see the problem.'
>
> G.K. Chesterton

PROBLEMS – FAMILIAR AND UNFAMILIAR

> 'Why is it so easy to acquire the solutions of past problems and so difficult to solve current ones?'
>
> Marshall McLuhan

Problems can be considered as a combination of familiar and unfamiliar tasks and familiar and unfamiliar settings, as shown in the Task/Setting matrix of Figure 16.

Figure 16 contains four cells:

In Cell 1: Someone remains in post within their present job and addresses a familiar issue. There is a continuing danger here that what has been chosen is either really a puzzle as opposed to a problem or has been contrived just for the purpose of the action learning programme – and so does not really embody the degree of challenge required.

In Cell 2: A person remains in their current job but tackles an issue which they have never previously addressed within that work role – something really novel and challenging.

In Cell 3: Someone takes on an issue with which they have previously had some success in their current job, but now they are faced with the challenge

		TASK	
		FAMILIAR	**UNFAMILIAR**
S E T T I N G	F a m i l i a r	1	2
	U n f a m i l i a r	3	4

Figure 16: Task/setting matrix

of trying to address this earlier success by tackling the same issue in another department, function or organisation, where they are not familiar with the history, culture and ways of working.

In Cell 4: Someone moves to another organisation or an unfamiliar part of their own organisation and tackles an unusual and previously unfamiliar problem.

Typically, the issues which set members are likely to address as part of an action learning programme will be those within their own job (Cell 1) or elsewhere within their own organisation (Cell 2). Action learning does not need to be confined to this focus, however. Many successful action learning programmes have been inter-organisational in both the private sector and between different parts of the public sector. For example, the former Scottish Leadership Foundation used inter-organisational action learning sets as part of its' work in developing collaborative working across public sector organisations (Cell 4). There is a strong case to be made for Cell 4 projects, although at first sight, it may seem counterintuitive. However, if the aim is to encourage the set member out of their comfort zone and to be placed in a situation where they must ask fresh questions and even challenge their own long-held assumptions, then Cell 4 is a powerful stimulus to learning.

Action learning set members can benefit from early focused thinking about whatever issue they wish to address in the set and in the workplace. Sometimes it can be difficult to choose across a range of possibilities. Using the Task/Setting Matrix in Figure 16 can help, as can the questions contained within the Action Learning Problem Brief shown in Table 5.

'If you think you understand a problem, make sure you are not deceiving yourself.'

Albert Einstein

Table 5: Action Learning Problem Brief

Describe your problem or issue in one sentence.
Why is this important to you? Why is it important to the organisation?
How will you recognise progress on the issue?
Who else would like to see progress on the issue?
How do you intend to go about tackling this problem? What will be your first steps?
What difficulties do you anticipate?
What will the benefits be to you and the organisation if this problem(s) is reduced or resolved?

'If you're not part of the problem, you can't be part of the solution.'

Adam Kahane

'A problem shared is a problem halved.'

Anon

REFERENCES

1. Garrat B. *The Learning Organisation*. London: Fontana-Collins; 1987.
2. Plsek P, Greenhalgh T. The challenge of complexity in health care. *BMJ*. 2004; **323**(7313): 625–28.
3. French R. Negative capability. In: Goethals G, Sorenson G, Burns J, editors. *Encyclopaedia of Leadership*. London: Sage; 2004.
4. Rittel H, Webber M. Dilemmas in a general theory of planning. *Policy Science*. 1973; **4**(1): 155–63.
5. Edmonstone J, Flanagan H. A flexible friend: action learning in the context of a multi-agency organisation development programme. *Action Learn Res Pract*. 2007; **4**(2): 199–209.

CHAPTER 6

Action learning sets

'We must indeed all hang together or, most assuredly, we shall all hang separately.'

Benjamin Franklin

Action learning sets are the main vehicle for learning and action and are central to how action learning works. They are concerned with:

➤ Helping set members to learn from the issues which they are addressing, so that they increasingly challenge their own and others' assumptions, review past actions, and their consequences, and plan the next stage.

➤ Implementing practical ways forward as well as diagnosing the nature of the problem.

➤ Moving into 'uncharted territory' where the issues are unfamiliar, rather than areas where set members already have experience.

Action learning sets are the means by which set members work out and pursue their own actions in the workplace and learn from that experience through the process of review, reflection and planning ahead.

PRINCIPLES FOR FORMING ACTION LEARNING SETS

Action learning offers a creative learning environment in which people can:

➤ Share insights and learn from each other.

➤ Create new links and strengthen existing relationships.

➤ Network and understand more about mutual roles and challenges – thus benefiting collaborative working.

➤ Provide space and time to consider work-related issues and come up with new ways of doing things.

The formation of action learning sets is, therefore, a vital process. There are a number of ways in which sets can be formed:

Set some criteria for the formation of sets

To help with the formation of sets, the facilitator could pre-determine some criteria to facilitate a discussion with potential set members about their own preferred criteria. The aim of such an approach would be to balance-out profession, role, background etc., of set members. This option might have the advantage of supporting broader learning by networking across a geographical 'patch'. Pre-determined criteria might include:

➤ *Geography* – for logistical travel and meeting purposes.
➤ *Gender mix* – a balance of male and female.
➤ *Diversity of personal style* – such as extrovert/introvert.
➤ *Mix of professional role and organisation* – for diversity of experience and background and to promote and enhance the potential for cross-system learning and networking.
➤ *Common areas of interest for addressing similar challenges* – although this may also limit the possible scope for learning.

Sets could be formed around a specific need such as, for people at a particular stage of their professional development or with similar developmental needs. While this would clearly be more tailored around individuals, it would perhaps not tap into the potential for local collaborative networking. This approach is relatively straightforward and manageable, but it does take away the element of choice on the part of potential set members, and may also lessen the learning, diversity and 'stretch' that may result from people forming their own sets.

Self-selection of set membership

With this approach, people are empowered to form their own sets. As such, it relies upon an iterative process within the group to arrive at flexible criteria for the self-selection of set members. For the approach to be relatively safe and productive, it is important to establish some clear ground-rules for set formation, such as:

➤ All sets must be **finally** formed at the same time.
➤ Conversations all take place in one room with everyone taking part.
➤ Sets need to be formed by the end of a set time period.

People must think about their own criteria for forming or joining a potential set and will need to engage in dialogue with other potential set members in arriving at set membership. A series of conversations (in pairs, trios and larger groups) across an agreed time-period can lead to the natural emergence of sets. The facilitator can help the process by suggesting questions which individuals might wish to address. These might include:

➤ Do I want to work with people I already know? Why?
➤ Should I seek to join a set with people I have never met? Why?
➤ Should I consider the professions/occupations of the other potential set members? Why?
➤ Should I aim to work with someone whose behaviour I find challenging?

What would be the advantages and disadvantages of this?
➤ Who will really challenge my thinking? Why?
➤ Are any potential set members' organisations/locations important to me?
➤ Does my project/challenge/issue have any implications for my choice? Why?

The advantage of this approach is that it can provide a powerful learning opportunity in its' own right – people start to create their own learning environment from the outset. However, it takes time and is likely to provoke feelings of anxiety and uncertainty for some people – the age-old feeling of 'Will I be picked for the team?'. Some people may even opt out of the process or dip in and out.

Whatever option for set formation is adopted there are four general criteria which remain critical when considering set membership. They are:

➤ *Interest*: Involvement in an action learning set should be voluntary wherever possible, not least because personal motivation plays an important role in sustaining effort on the part of the set member over the life of the set. Potential set members should recognise that a problem or issue exists, should want to tackle it and should see the set as a useful support in doing so.

➤ *Diversity*: The personal skills and qualities of set members, together with their different professional, departmental and organisational experiences and styles all come together to create a 'rich mixture' for the set. Sufficient contrast is required to provide the 'grit in the oyster' of the set, but with the obvious danger that too great a diversity may also create problems and the set may find it difficult to develop a shared sense of identity. With a diverse set membership, an 'unfamiliarity factor' becomes embedded. Diversity necessitates having to deal with other age groups, gender, cultures, etc., – all of which can serve to enrich the dialogue and open up new ways of seeing and understanding. Diversity, however, needs to be balanced with equality (see below).

➤ *Equality*: It can help if the set shares a broadly common age range and/ or work experience, together with roughly the same level of career progression and achievement. The intellectual and emotional capacity of set members should be generally similar because it is important that no set member ever feels out of their depth.

➤ *Level of Challenge*: The challenge inherent in the issue chosen should be broadly similar for all set members. Issues chosen should:
  – Be real and significant, both for the individual and the organisation.
  – Involve action as well as diagnosis.
  – Not have been previously addressed.
  – Be defined in some way (tightly or loosely).
  – Be capable of being learned from.

It is sensible not to have people with a history of personal animosity as members of the same set. Action learning is not meant to be a means of conflict resolution! People who 'have a history' between them are unlikely to feel safe in each other's company, and are likely to colour the tone of other set members' involvement. Moreover, they are less likely to open themselves up for deeper exploration of the issues they bring to the set.

Alternative set groupings

Sets should comprise around a maximum of seven or eight people. More than eight, and some of the free and spontaneous interaction that marks set meetings, is impossible. Eight diaries also make agreeing dates for meetings a nightmare. There are three alternative configurations or set groupings. These are:

➤ *Vertical sets*: These are sets made up of members drawn from different levels within the same profession, function or department. This type of set shows evidence of strong support and commitment from the profession or department, and promotes the concept of equality of contribution from all individuals. This kind of grouping allows a full spectrum of views and opinions on particular issues and provides a ready-made means of communication between all the grades and levels concerned, so the likelihood of action is much more certain. However, if there are over-hierarchical or dominant relationships already in existence, then such groupings may only serve to stifle the input of set members. Difficulties in communicating ideas and concerns may also occur, due to differences in both perspective and ability.

➤ *Horizontal sets*: These are made up of people working at a similar level within one, or across a number of, organisations – and, as such, is the configuration adopted by the majority of sets. Shared experience and common ground can help to reduce barriers quickly and encourage greater levels of trust. The set members may find it easier to establish agreed social processes and feel more comfortable in offering spirited challenge to each other. On the other hand, if people's perspectives are fairly familiar and set members are happy with these established patterns, then it may be more difficult to shake or challenge shared views. In such circumstances, any power games between set members may be quite subtle, difficult to spot and tricky to deal with.

➤ *Combination sets*: These involve mixing these two major types together.

➤ *Hybrid sets:* When there is a number of action learning sets running across an organisation or organisations, then there may be advantage in also creating another set made up of members of the 'regular' sets to focus on what learning is taking place across the whole system, rather than the more specific issues which set members are addressing.

There may be occasions where such is the relative 'immaturity' within the potential overall set membership (manifested in significant diversity and/or stereotyping) that there may be a case for forming discrete and 'identifiable' sets in the first instance, thus giving set members the space to first come together and establish a sense of identity, before then forming 'mixed' sets made up out of the earlier groupings – a process of integration before differentiation.

Question regarding set membership

There are some questions which are worth asking by organisations and facilitators when thinking about the potential membership of a set. They include:

➤ Is there anyone missing who could really contribute to the life of the set?
➤ Will everyone who is interested in being a set member be allowed to attend set meetings or will they be subject to pressure or criticism from their boss and/or colleagues for doing so?
➤ Will the configurations produce all-female, all-male or mixed gender sets? Does it matter?
➤ What will be the maximum and minimum number of members in the set?
➤ Who is it important to have in the sets?

The answers to these questions will vary according to the focus of the sets and the overall intentions of the action learning programme.

There is also a question regarding the consistency of likely involvement in the set. It is often impossible, due to staffing pressures and family commitments, for every set member to attend every set meeting, but more than one absence of any one member can hold back the effectiveness of the set. Asking potential set members to identify potential pressures on set members at the outset can be a useful 'screening' activity.

Agreeing set ground-rules

Early in the life of any set, there will be a need to establish ground-rules to govern the behaviour of set members and the facilitator; to allay any fears people may have about what might happen in the set, and to establish and model shared responsibility and joint working between the set members and the facilitator. These ground rules make it far less likely that set members will be disappointed or frustrated by the behaviour of the other members of the set. Ground-rules are of two types.

Practical ground-rules cover such matters as:

➤ The life-expectancy of the set – how long will it continue to meet?
➤ The frequency and duration of set meetings – how often will the set meet and for how long on each occasion?
➤ The format of meetings and how time will be allocated within them.

Behavioural ground-rules need to address such matters as:

➤ *Commitment and priority*: Set members will be busy people with multiple calls on their time. To attend set meetings and to engage fully in the life of the set takes a degree of commitment, and an agreement to make both set meetings as well as the work-based activity that occurs between them a priority, is vital. This requires self-discipline among set members and it is important to address these issues right at the start of the set's life. One practical example of such self-discipline would involve all set members agreeing to turn off their mobile phones for the duration of all set meetings.

➤ *Confidentiality*: While all set members are likely to subscribe to the principle of confidentiality, it is an important job for the facilitator, at an early stage, to help the set members to tease out exactly what is meant in practice by this term. Confidentiality can never be absolute, so the aim should be to establish the limits of confidentiality and to agree on any circumstances when set members and the facilitator might communicate information to people outside the set. For example, a set member may ask for support or advice from another set member between meetings. It is most important that these circumstances are clear to every set member, as this allows them to make an informed choice about exactly what they disclose in the set.

➤ *Timekeeping:* To ensure that each set member has a fair share of the time available for their issue, it will be important to keep to both the external time-boundaries of the set meeting (which means starting and finishing on time), as well as the internal time-boundaries (the amount of time allocated in a set meeting to each set member).

➤ *Equal Airtime*: For the duration of any one set member's airtime, the other set members are there to listen and to enable the focal set member in working on the issue or problem they are addressing. If the focal set member is not receiving the kind of help needed, then he or she should say so. It will be important to avoid the use of anecdotes or dwelling on other set members' parallel issues, so danger signs would be hearing set members say *'I have a similar problem with my staff.'*, *'I had difficulties with her when she worked for me.'* or *'We all know what he's like!'.*

➤ *Only One Person Speaks At A Time:* There should be no 'talking-over' or interrupting the contributions of other set members.

➤ *'I' Language:* Set members need to use the word *'I'* instead of *'one'*, *'we'*, *'you'* or *'they'*, as it helps them get closer to the problem situation.

➤ *Openness:* The success of the set will depend to a great extent on the degree to which set members feel comfortable enough to be open with each other.

➤ *Enabling Behaviour*: The other set members are there to help the set member to focus on his or her issue, in order to find the best possible course of action, not to offer their own solutions, unless requested to do so by the focal set member or as part of a brainstorm of possibilities. It has been suggested that:

'Only in a group where it is safe to disclose ignorance, admit weakness and ask for help, is it possible for the problem-holder to learn at sufficient depth for him or her to develop as an individual.'[1]

➤ The set should provide a safe and experimental space where each set member can take the risk of trying-out new ways of relating to others, knowing that they will get constructive feedback and not be blamed for 'getting it wrong'.

Ground-rules for an action learning set might look something like those shown in Table 6.

Table 6: Action Learning Set Ground-rules

Each person will turn up on time.
Meetings will start and finish on time.
Each person will let the others know if they cannot attend a meeting.
If a person says that something is confidential then it will not be discussed outside the set.
Each person's contribution shall be valued.
No person's ideas will be ridiculed.
No one person will dominate the conversation.
Each person will contribute at least one thing to each meeting.
Each person will have done any agreed work between meetings.
Each person will come to the set meeting prepared.

The precise number of ground-rules decided upon by the set members is not important and will vary from set to set. It is more important to establish five ground-rules that all set members agree to stick to than twenty-five that they will not! The most important ground-rule is the one that says that all ground-rules are open to renegotiation and that new ground-rules can be agreed at any time the set feels it is necessary.

A useful process for creating ground-rules is:
➤ Seek suggestions from set members.
➤ Encourage debate about what they mean.
➤ Write-up the agreed ground-rules on a flipchart.
➤ Either post the flipchart at every set meeting in full view of set members, or have the ground-rules e-mailed to all set members, or both.

➤ Point out that ground-rules can be added to or renegotiated as the life of the set develops.

➤ Use the ground-rules as part of the review process at the end of the set meeting.[2]

LOCATION AND VENUE OF SET MEETINGS

Where the set meets is important and will clearly depend upon geography, travel times and distances. A quiet, adequately-heated and well-ventilated room is the basic requirement. The seating should be comfortable and, if possible, the chairs should be of the same design and arranged in a circle or rectangle. Tea- and coffee-making facilities and eating arrangements must be clear and flipchart pads and pens, etc., should be easily available. In the early stages of the set's life, the facilitator may take responsibility for such matters, but as the set develops the set members should increasingly take over this responsibility.

When set meetings take place in work organisations, there is always the possibility of interruptions, so an early ground-rule covering this eventuality may be necessary. Alternatively, the set might opt for a less convenient, but 'neutral', venue to which some of the set members have to travel, and which might, therefore, involve extra cost. Should the set involve people based in a variety of locations, then there may be value in moving the venue around for each set meeting, so that each set member takes it in turn to act as host or hostess – but beware competition over provision of lunches!

In thinking about the venue of set meetings, the issue of boundary protection is important. This means ensuring set members feel they are operating in a safe and supportive environment where they can feel OK about addressing their work-related concerns. The set acts as a holding environment or transitional space in which set members can handle their anxiety. So, the extent to which the set is able to exclude the immediate demands and pressures of the set members' work environments and create a space which is truly the set's own for the duration of the set meeting, without any intrusion of work pressures, is likely to be key to success.

FREQUENCY OF SET MEETINGS

Action learning sets typically run from a minimum of six months to one year or more, but there does need to be a clearly-defined end-point. The gap between set meetings should not be so close that the time commitment and attendance are problematic – especially when challenging action on individual issues is required in between meetings – and not too far apart for set members to lose the thread of what is happening. Meetings often take place every four to six weeks. All meetings need to be planned and booked well in advance – in diaries and personal organisers – from the first, start-up meeting. Key holiday periods should be taken into account to ensure maximum attendance levels.

DURATION OF SET MEETINGS

The larger the set membership, the longer the set meeting will need to last – or alternatively, the more truncated the individual time-slots for set members will be. An action learning set should, as a broad rule-of-thumb, allow at least forty-five minutes per participant at each meeting, and if there are more than four participants, it is wise to add at least thirty minutes for slippage or for comfort breaks within the session. No set is entirely 'typical' but, on average, a set of five members might well last for three to four hours, while a set of seven members would probably last a whole day.

WHAT HAPPENS IN THE SET

> 'Coming together is the beginning. Keeping together is progress. Working together is success.'
>
> Henry Ford

There are a number of major activities which take place in a set meeting:
➤ Set members share their viewpoints on the issues being addressed.
➤ They support and challenge each other in developing a better understanding of a problem situation, through questioning their own and each other's perceptions, in developing the insight that results from this process and in identifying possible actions.
➤ The set develops over time – it forms, matures and learns how to work together productively and creatively.
➤ The set members review and evaluate how well the set is operating.

Set meetings therefore usually go through a number of stages:
➤ *Catching-Up or 'What's On Top?'* This serves to allow set members to check-in, to say where they are at personally, and to share their immediate 'hot' news. It helps to reintroduce and reintegrate the set, build or rebuild the group identity and keep the set rooted in what the world is like 'out there'. Sometimes a warm-up exercise might be used for the same purpose, especially in the early days of the set.
➤ *Agenda-Setting*: In many instances, this will involve simply confirming the format agreed at the last set meeting, or modifying it by agreement. In other cases, the set members will agree the agenda and running-order and allocate the time available. While a basic premise of set meetings is that all set members have equal 'airtime', this may be modified by agreement, depending on need or urgency.
➤ *Progress-Reporting*: Each set member has a time-slot and takes it in turn to report on progress made with their issue since the last set meeting; the current state of play. The more set members can think things through in advance of set meetings, structure their time well within their time-slot, specify clearly what they want the set members to focus on, ask for what

they want and conclude by generating actions for themselves, then the more they will benefit from the work of the set.

Set members have a range of options for how they might use their time-slot. They might, for example:

➤ Ask other set members to listen while they give a short presentation and then ask for comments. They might have a pre-prepared flipchart or handout listing the key points they want to address, or present them on a flipchart in real time. If they do this, they then talk, without interruption, for as long as they wish, about the situation.

➤ Ask for questions from the other set members which are designed to help the individual concerned come to a deeper understanding of their issue.

➤ Ask the other set members to brainstorm ways of tackling a problem which they currently face.

➤ Request the other set members to discuss the question they have presented while:

  – They, themselves, take personal notes of useful ideas that may emerge.
  – Tape-record their time-slot and replay it later.
  – Review and record options, then decide on action.

The set meeting thus focuses on each set member and their issue in turn, supporting, challenging and questioning – and also offering resources of various kinds – contacts, materials, sources and so on, with set members helping the person with the issue to learn from what has happened and to find a way forward. People bring the whole of themselves to the process of the set and have the freedom to explore as much as they feel comfortable with, without making a rigid boundary between work and non-work issues.

As the set progresses, the balance of time devoted to different activities changes. Time spent on describing or reporting on the problem or issue declines, as does time spent on clarifying the problem. With the passage of time more and more time is devoted to attempts at resolution of the problem and to practical actions in the workplace, as is shown in Figure 17.

➤ *Review:* At the end of each set meeting some time for reflection, feedback and discussion on individual and group processes is valuable. It should concentrate on such questions as *'What worked well today?'*, *'Was there a problem with this meeting?'* or *'How can we be more effective next time?'*

'It can be no dishonour to learn from others, when they speak good sense.'

Sophocles

TIME AND PROCESS

Most members come to set meetings straight from a work environment where the norm is to 'shoot from the hip' in addressing problems. The learned instinct

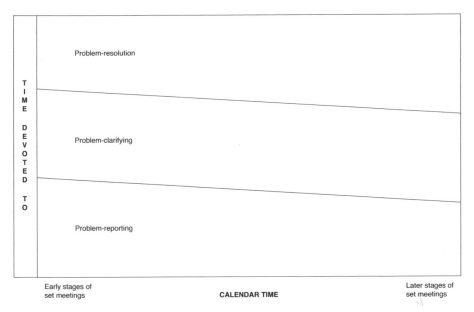

Figure 17: Time-distribution of activities within action learning sets

at work is to troubleshoot and fix things – to break down the ambiguity, resolve the paradox, achieve greater certainty and agreement and be seduced by instant solutions. To this, could also be added the often-frenzied intensity and repetitiveness of daily work events. Bringing a problem to the set; explaining it in sufficient depth as to be helpful; allowing questioning and reflection; exploring new ideas – all of these take time and involve slowing-down. This can be a liberating experience, but can be such a contrast to the world of work that there is a danger of trying to change the tempo of the set to match that of the work environment. This must be resisted. For some set members, the ability to reflect may be undeveloped, so that when they attempt it they may feel extremely awkward – like a right-handed person trying to sign their name with their left hand. It takes time and practice to unlock the ability to reflect. The Break-Space Exercise in Part 3 of this book can help to aid the reflective process.

Action learning fosters dialogue rather than debate. The origin of the word debate means to 'beat down'. The word dialogue comes from the Greek 'dia-logos' meaning 'to hang from'. This distinction is important – in action learning, dialogue offers a chance to respect, question, consider and apply different contributions, by allowing them time to 'hang'. Argument and debate (the beating-down of ideas), by contrast, allows little time or respect for others and has a competitive edge – coming-up with the 'best' idea or 'trumping' another's contribution.

Table 7 suggests that a high degree of tolerance for fellow set members is crucial here. The table can be a useful aid for creating and encouraging tolerance within the set.

Table 7: Different drums and different drummers

If I do not want what you want, please do not try to tell me what I want is wrong.
Or, if I believe other than you, at least pause before you correct my view.
Or, if my emotion is less than yours, or more, given the same circumstances, try not to ask me to feel more strongly or weakly.
Or, yet if I act, or fail to act, in the manner of your design for action, let me be.
I do not, for the moment at least, ask you to understand me. That will come only when you are willing to give up changing me into a copy of you.

'Alone we can do so little; together we can do so much.'

Helen Keller

SUPPORT AND CHALLENGE

'Trust is the bandwidth of communication.'

Karl-Erik Sveiby

At the heart of set meetings, are the twin activities of support and challenge. Support (or emotional warmth) cannot be simply 'engineered' and may take time to build, although the facilitator (and set members) can certainly accelerate the process. An appropriate degree of support is often needed before real challenge can be acceptable. Too much challenge, especially too early, can be experienced by set members as stressful and counter-productive, but too little is also unhelpful. Balancing support and challenge is important and helps the learning process, as is shown in Figure 18.

It is possible to assess the degree of support and challenge that each set member has felt they received during the set meeting by using a simple Support/Challenge Map, as shown in the Resources section in Part 3 of this book.

Appropriate attitudes and behaviour

Within sets, therefore, it is possible to highlight what are appropriate attitudes and behaviour. Helpful attitudes include:

➤ *Concern for the well-being of other set members*: All set members need to care sufficiently about their colleagues to want them to succeed with their issue and to learn from the experience.

➤ *Each set member is the expert on their own problem:* The person asking the question or addressing the issue will always have access to information which they might not, either by choice or circumstance, share with other set members. So only by believing that people can help themselves, can effective help really be given. Respect is therefore needed for the judgement of other set members in identifying what they do and do not choose to share in the set's discussion.

High Challenge & Low Support	Sufficient Challenge & Support
Increased stress Feels competitive & critical Disempowering	Motivational Developmental
Low Challenge & Low Support	Too Much Support & Low Challenge
Boring Distant Absent Avoidance	Stifling Controlling Patronising

Figure 18: Balancing support and challenge

➤ *Empathy*: A willingness to share the feelings and thoughts of someone else – to ask yourself *'What does it feel like to be that person with that problem?'* – an attitude which is both thoughtful and curious about the person with the problem – a type of 'intelligent naivety'.

Derived from these attitudes, helpful behaviours include:
➤ *Challenging* – by questioning.
➤ *Supporting* – providing assistance in both the set meetings and between them (by telephone, e-mail, providing contacts, material, etc.)
➤ *Conveying empathy* – a powerful means of giving the person with the problem permission to share more.
➤ *Learning not to interrupt* – jotting-down emerging thoughts and ideas in order to contribute later.
➤ *Active listening* (to what set members say and don't say) and *attending* (to non-verbal cues) will ensure full and close attention.
➤ Continually asking *'Is this helpful?'*.

So, it is possible to say that the attributes of being an effective set member are:[3]
➤ Being willing to attend to others when it is their turn to present their issue.
➤ Actively listening and not talking-over other people.
➤ Allowing time for others to reflect and not always filling a silence.
➤ Allowing the person to present their own issue and, at the same time, avoiding passing judgement or offering solutions.
➤ Being prepared to commit to being an active set member for the duration of the set's life.

➤ Attempting to undertake the actions agreed at the end of the personal time-slot.

➤ Reflecting on personal progress and plans, in order to learn from the experience.

➤ Trusting the overall process and acting within it in good faith.

➤ Collaborating with others in the set to make it work as well for all members.

Experience can be a very 'slippery' teacher – most of the time we have experiences from which we seldom learn. Action learning seeks to throw a net around slippery experiences and capture them as learning – by encouraging reflection, promoting insightful inquiry and leaving responsibility for taking action firmly with the set member.

Between set meetings: preparing for the next time

To get the most out of action learning, it is necessary for set members to do some preparation for a set meeting. The most important preparation any set member can do is obviously to take all the actions that they agreed to do at the previous set meeting!

In addition to this, there are some questions which a set member can usefully think about in preparation:

➤ What have I done since the last set meeting?

➤ Are there still some outstanding action points that I have not pursued? What are they? Why have I not pursued them?

➤ Do I still see the issue or problem in the same way as I did originally?

➤ What have I learned so far from what I've done? – about myself; others; the issue or problem.

➤ How have my plans changed since the last set meeting? Why?

➤ What are my next steps?

➤ What do I need from this next set meeting?

➤ How can my fellow set members help me?

'One must be fond of people and trust them if one is not to make a mess of life.'

E.M. Forster

REFERENCES

1. Gaunt R, Kendall R. *Action Learning: a short manual for set members*. London: Greater London Employers Secretariat; 1985.
2. Havergal M, Edmonstone J. *The Facilitator's Toolkit*. Aldershot: Gower Publishing; 2003.
3. Beaty L. *Action Learning*. York: Learning Teacher Support Network, CPD Paper No. 1; 2003.

CHAPTER 7

Listening and questioning: the key skills

'"Forty-two!" yelled Loonquawl. "Is that all you've got to show from seven and a half million years' work?" "I checked it very thoroughly," said the computer, "and that quite definitely is the answer. I think the problem, to be quite honest with you, is that you've never really known what the question is......Once you know what the question is, you'll know what the answer means."'

Douglas Adams – The Hitchhiker's Guide to the Galaxy

ACTIVE LISTENING

'Conversation doesn't just reshuffle the cards. It creates new cards.'

Theodore Zeldin

Actively listening to the other set members enables each person to:
➤ Learn about their needs and wants.
➤ Understand what motivates them.
➤ Make them feel valued.
➤ Build trust and rapport.

The purpose of active listening is to allow the other set member to express his or her self, as fully and openly as possible. It enables them to 'think aloud' in order to solve their own problem, or to be properly heard and understood, so that they can let a situation go and move on. There are four steps for active listening:

1. *Listening*: This is not as simple an activity as most people think. It is not just a person sitting and looking as if they are listening, while composing what they intend to say next. Instead, it involves listening with real attention to try to understand the thoughts and feelings of the other person and why they think and feel like they do, without wanting to change them. It is the:

    'ability of the listener to capture and understand the messages communicated by the presenter, whether these messages are transmitted verbally or non-verbally, clearly or vaguely.'[1]

➤ Some hints for effective active listening are:
  – You have two ears and one mouth – use them in that proportion!
  – As far as possible, sit facing the set member with a posture that conveys involvement. Look interested and stay alert.
  – Adopt an open posture – crossed arms or legs may convey a closed stance. Maintain eye contact with the set member.
  – Minimise distractions.
  – Don't fidget or play with pens. Retain a reasonable level of eye contact. Sit upright and look attentive.
  – Make notes if you want to remember something. It also shows interest, provided you don't look down too much.
  – You need to stop your thoughts or pause internal 'self-talk' in order to pay attention. One way of doing this is to repeat what the other set member is saying in your mind a fraction of a second after they say it. Do not try and plan what you intend to say next.
  – Check-out whether the set member is triggering feelings and memories within yourself that are more 'yours' than theirs. If they are, try not to react to them.
  – Attend to more than the set member's words – take note of their language, tone of voice and expression, as well as their body language.
  – Don't leap in and interrupt with personal stories of similar experiences. Listen without interruption – take your cue from the set member before intervening.
  – Leave pauses and allow for silence – although most people feel uncomfortable with this and seek to fill the gaps with words, the set member may require time to think internally and privately. Also, important information often comes in the afterthought, so never finish people's sentences.

2. *Paraphrasing:* Use at least some of the set member's own words and metaphors to let them know that you have heard them. Sometimes people are quite surprised about what they have said and it can be very powerful to have it reflected back to them.

3. *Checking Understanding*: Be curious and do not assume that you have necessarily understood what the set member has said. It is very easy to impose our own frame of reference. So, if they say, for example *'I feel bad'* then respond with *'Bad – like what?'.*

4. *Suspending Judgement*: Be assured that the set member has a reason for their particular perspective and that they want to work things out and move forward. They are capable of addressing their own problems, given time and the opportunity to think things through. Do not jump in to 'fix' problems – it's very disrespectful and disempowering and you are probably doing it more for your own benefit than for theirs.

Table 8 is a helpful aide memoire.

Table 8: Listen

> When I ask you to listen to me and you give me advice, you have not done what I asked.
>
> When I ask you to listen to me and you feel you have to do something to solve my problems, you have failed me, strange as that may seem.
>
> Listen! All I asked was that you listen. Not talk or do – just hear me. Advice is cheap. Look in any cheap newspaper and you will find several different kinds of advice.
>
> And, I can do for myself – I'm not helpless.
>
> When you do something for me, that I can and need to do for myself, you contribute to my fear and weakness.
>
> But, when you accept as a simple fact that I do feel what I feel, no matter how irrational, then I stop trying to convince you and can get back to the business of understanding what may be behind these irrational feelings.
>
> And, when that's clear, the answers are obvious and I don't need advice.
>
> Irrational feelings make sense when we understand what's behind them.
>
> So, please listen and just hear me, and, if you want to talk, wait a minute for your turn, and I'll listen to you.
>
> Anon

Active listening can be hampered by:
➤ *Evaluative listening* – when we impose our own values on the set member's message, judging what we are hearing whilst it is being transmitted instead of putting thoughts to one side to hear what is truly being conveyed.
➤ *Comparison* – when we are comparing ourselves to the set member speaking.
➤ *Inattentive listening* – when we are distracted by other things, our tiredness or our own emotions.
➤ *Thinking how to respond* – a listener who is preoccupied with their own response to the set member may stop listening to, and therefore attending to, the set member.
➤ *Second guessing* – and not just allowing the set member who is speaking to unfold at their own pace.
➤ *Listening with sympathy rather than empathy* – by offering our sympathy at feelings of loss or sorrow, we may get in the way of helping the set member to move on. Empathy is the ability to observe and not absorb, so that we can respond and not react to the set member.

QUESTIONING

> 'My mother made me a scientist without ever intending to. Every other Jewish mother in Brooklyn would ask her child after school "So, did you learn anything today?" But not my mother. "Izzy" she would say, "did you ask a good question today?"'
>
> Isidor Isaac Rabi

Insightful questioning clearly grows out of active listening – the quality of the questions asked is a function of our ability to listen effectively. Questions aim to enable the set member to broaden or deepen their view of the situation or issue they are addressing and to take responsibility for themselves to work through it, rather than being given 'solutions' – which is disempowering. Good questions come from a deep interest in the set member's experience – they offer the set member the chance to ponder further. The aim is to tap into our own different view of the world **only in order to enhance or extend the set member's view of themselves and their situation.**

Argyris and Schon[2] have identified what they call Model I and Model II approaches to questioning, as shown in Table 9.

Table 9: Two Models Of Questioning

Model I	Model II
Asking questions in such a way as to get the other person to agree with one's view.	Actively inquiring into the other's views and the reasoning that supports them.
Advocating one's own view in a manner that limits others' questioning of it.	Advocating one's view and reasoning in a way that encourages others to confront it and to help the speaker discover where the view may be mistaken.
Privately evaluating the other person's view and attributing causes to it.	Stating publicly the inferences that one makes about others and the data that leads to those inferences, and inviting others to correct the inferences if they are inaccurate.

We tend to use Model I behaviours in our day-to-day interactions but action learning creates the opportunity to use Model II behaviour.

Revans suggested there were three major questions which every set member needed to pose in relation to the issue they were addressing. They were:

1. *Who knows?* Who has useful information? – the hard facts that will determine the dimensions of the problem, and not official policies, opinions, personal views or half-truths.
2. *Who cares?* Who has the emotional investment and energy to mobilise change? Who is involved and committed to an outcome, rather than who just talks about the issue?

3. **Who can?** Who has the power to allocate or reallocate resources so that change can happen? Who, when faced with the facts, commitment and energy, has the power to say *'Yes'*?

These questions relate to three crucial processes in human action – thinking, feeling and willing. Most of our formal educational system concentrates on the first question and on the thinking process (*see* Chapter 2). Yet, the degree of emotional commitment (feeling) and power (willing) that exists is also important. If the concentration is on thinking alone then there is a danger of 'paralysis-by-analysis' where diagnosis and planning never lead to action.

The importance of these three questions can be shown by use of the ***Thinking, Feeling & Willing Exercise*** in Part 3 of this book.

It has also been suggested that other major questions which can be posed as part of the process of action learning are:

What is it that you do? What is the nature of your work, role or task?

What are you trying to do? What is driving you? What is your motivation?

What's stopping you? What are the blockages or obstructions?

Who and what can help you? What are the resources you need to draw on or mobilise?

Questions asked by set members and the facilitator can be both helpful and unhelpful. Helpful questions include:

➤ *Open questions* aimed at stimulating an extended free response. These are questions that begin with *'What'*, *'Where'*, *'Which'*, *'Why'*, *'How'* and *'When'.*

➤ *Awareness-raising questions* like *'How did you feel when you were involved in that?'* or *'What do you imagine it would look like if you were to do it differently?'* Such questions encourage self-awareness and focus on positive ideas for future action.

➤ *Elaborating questions* that give the set member an opportunity to expand on what they have already started to describe. Examples include *'Could you say a little more about that?'* and *'Could you elaborate on what you just said?'*

➤ *Reflective questions* help to get clarification by 'replaying' the set member's words or re-phrasing them and reflecting them back in order to test understanding and to encourage the set member to talk more. Examples are: *'So what you seem to be saying is …'* or *'Let me just check I'm understanding you correctly…'*

➤ *Specification questions* aim to get more detail out about the problem situation by asking things like *'When you say she angers you, what exactly happens?'*

➤ *Justifying questions* provide an opportunity for the set member to further explain their reasons attitudes or feelings. Examples are *'How would you explain that to someone else?'* or *'Could you help me to understand you by putting it another way?'*

➤ *Focusing on feelings questions* aim to tease out the emotions linked to the issue which the set member is addressing. Such questions should be tentative since the set member should know their own feelings better than anyone else. Examples would be *'How do you feel about that?'* and *'I seem to hear you saying that you feel ….'*

➤ *Personal ownership questions* imply not only that the set member has a responsibility for owning the issue, but also for making the choices that contribute to moving it forward. Such questions aim to make links between how the set member describes the issue initially and their role in sustaining or resolving it.

➤ Examples are *'How do you see your own behaviour contributing to this situation?'* and *'Are there ways in which you might be helping yourself more?'*

➤ *Hypothetical questions* pose a situation or suggestion – a *'What if?'* or *'How about?'* and can be useful for introducing a new idea or challenging a response.

➤ *Checking questions* like *'Is this always true in every situation?'* check what is being heard or correct understanding.

➤ *Incisive questions* come in two parts. The first part asserts a positive assumption while the second directs the set member's attention back to the need for action. Examples include *'If you were told that your future job prospects depended on changing the way you worked, what would you do first?'*, *'If you were in charge, what would you tackle first and how would you go about it?'* and *'If things were exactly right for you in this situation, how would they have changed?'*

The aim is always to find and use those questions which encourage the set member to question themselves – the process which fosters questioning insight. A good question is selfless. It is not asked in order to highlight how clever the questioner is or to generate more information for the questioner – rather it is a means of opening-up the set member's own view of the issue or problem.

An opportunity it try-out questioning is contained in the *Slow-Motioning Questioning Exercise* in Part 3 of this book.

In contrast, unhelpful questions include:

➤ *Closed questions* that can only be answered by *'Yes'* or *'No'*, and which curtail the set member's options for responding. They usually begin with a *'Do you…?'*, and *'Are you …?'* or *'Have you …?'* Closed questions can, on occasion, have positive uses, when they are used as a challenge, as in *'Do you **really** want to do anything about this?'*

➤ *Leading or loaded questions* put the answer into the set member's mouth and usually demonstrate what the person asking them already knows (or think they know) rather than what the set member really understands or believes.

➤ *Multiple questions*, or several question rolled into one mean that the set member will inevitably choose the easiest question and avoid the difficult one that is part of the same 'package'.

➤ *Long-winded questions* will probably be misunderstood.

➤ *Overly-probing questions* – those the set member is not yet ready to answer, given the level of trust in the set.

➤ *Poorly-timed questions* interrupt the set member from working on the issue themselves and come at the wrong point in the helping process.

➤ *Trick questions* are likely to cause resentment, de-motivation and even withdrawal.

➤ *Too many questions* will feel like an interrogation and lead to defensiveness.

There are some useful questions which each set member can ask themselves in preparation for their part of a set meeting and these are shown in Table 10.

Table 10: Preparatory questions for set members

What am I trying to do?
What's stopping me from doing it?
How do I feel about that?
What can I do about it?
Who knows what I'm trying to do? Who has the necessary information?
Who cares about what I'm trying to do? Who feel emotionally involved?
Who can do anything to help? Who has the 'clout' to make a difference?
What has happened since the last set meeting? What have I done?
What has been different from what I expected?
What did I not do and why?
What did I do instead and why?
What would a positive outcome look like?
What have I (or can I) learn from this?

Similarly, there are questions which set members and the facilitator might want to use to help the person with the issue or problem and these are shown in Table 11.

Table 11: Question for use by set members and facilitator

Questions for focusing attention on the present situation
What's important to you about this issue and why do you care?
What are the dilemmas/opportunities in relation to this issue?
What is important in dealing with this issue – what people expect of you or what you expect of yourself?
What do you do well in your current job and what do others see that you do well? How can these be best used in tackling this issue?
What are your unique contributions to enable this issue to be tackled effectively?
Questions for reviewing future possibilities:
What assumptions do you need to test or challenge about dealing with this issue?
What challenges are raised that you really look forward to – or prefer to avoid?
What support can you call upon to encourage you as you face the change issues?
Questions that create movement towards new possibilities:
What needs your priority and attention going forward?
How can you get the support needed in taking the next steps?
What is needed to give you the confidence to move forward successfully?
What is it that you fear? How can you allay this fear?

Set members may sometimes need help in translating the issue or problem they face into a challenge. There is therefore a need to move from a focus on the problem to one where the focus is on *'How can I ....?* The following questions can help this transition:

➤ What exactly are you trying to do?
➤ What's stopping you from doing it?
➤ Who can help you to do it?
➤ What do you need to be able to know or do in order to do it?

> 'Through constant questioning we see more clearly just who we really are and what remarkable resources we have access to. We will also see more clearly what is really facing us and will become more capable of accepting and responding to change.'
>
> Reg Revans

REFERENCES

1. Egan G. *The Skilled Helper: a problem-management approach to helping.* Belmont, CA: Brooks-Cole Publishing; 1993.
2. Argyris C, Schon D. *Organisational Learning II.* Reading, MA: Addison-Wesley; 1996.

CHAPTER 8

And other skills

A range of challenges face people who become the members of an action learning set. They include the challenges of:

➤ Learning to cope without a trainer (i.e., not being taught).
➤ Linking learning with work.
➤ Learning from colleagues.
➤ Reflecting (in order to make sense of experience)
➤ Keeping going (over an extensive period, often with gaps between face-to-face meetings).

LEARNING TO COPE WITHOUT A TRAINER

For many set members, being a member of an action learning set can be a strange experience. Their typical experience will be sitting in a training centre or classroom with other learners and a trainer. In the action learning set, some of these features are repeated – but the 'trainer' doesn't teach them anything! This problem can be addressed by acknowledging the likely feelings of discomfort; by structuring the equal time-sharing for set members; by the facilitator emphasising a willingness to co-operatively support the overall learning process, and by encouraging the taking of first steps.

LINKING LEARNING WITH WORK

'The work will teach you how to do it.'

Estonian proverb

For many people the world of work and the world of learning are not linked. The former is the arena of acting and doing, while the latter is concerned with reflecting and conceptualising.[1] The choice of the project or issue by set members and their sponsors within their organisations can help to link these two spheres. If the area chosen is too much like ordinary work, then it may not be seen as a source of rich learning. If it is too untypical of ordinary work, then it may not be seen as relevant, although that will depend on the ability of the set member to conceptualise the linkages between work and learning. The facilitator and other set members have a key role to play here, but other things which can help include ensuring that the issues chosen have an inter-professional or inter-organisational focus; ensuring that front-line clinical staff have to interact with senior managers to pursue their issue or question and by requiring contact to address the topic with service-users and carers.

> 'The future of work consists of learning a living.'
>
> Marshall McLuhan

LEARNING FROM COLLEAGUES

While Revans called set members 'comrades in adversity', other things can also help the process of learning from colleagues. One is the notion of needs and offers. At the beginning of an action learning programme, (and at intervals during the programme) there can be value in asking set members to write down what they want and what they have to offer – and then to post the results on a flipchart for all set members to see. This process can lead to person-to-person linkages of the kind *'I see you need to know more about process mapping. I did a workshop on this a few months ago and applied it with my staff – I'd be happy to talk it through with you.'* However, it can take some time for this process to get going as people can feel 'selfish' in addressing their own hopes and fears, and may believe that this cannot possibly be enriching and illuminating for their fellow set members.

If the set members are only writing down notes from what the facilitator is saying, the facilitator may want to point this out to them!

> 'All learning is for the sake of action, and all action is for the sake of friendship.'
>
> John MacMurray

REFLECTING

As the set gets going, the facilitator role (and that of the set members) tends to move from energising and speeding things up, to reflecting and slowing things down. This can involve not only asking set members to work together in pairs and reviewing achievements to date, but also in encouraging set members to take responsibility for their actions; and to seeing themselves as the cause of what happens to them; not blaming themselves for these actions and finally, to enhancing their learning by generalising from their experience.

KEEPING GOING

Energy levels in action learning sets can vary. Sometimes set members can be 'fired-up' and involved but, on other occasions, they can wilt and a sense of hopelessness can develop. The set facilitator should be sensitive to these mood changes but should simply reflect on what they see, rather than trying to 'lift' the set. However, other things that can help to develop a sense of stamina for the set include:

➤ Sharing telephone numbers and e-mail addresses so that set members can check-out each other's progress.

➤ Encouraging set members to meet in pairs and trios between agreed set meetings.

➤ Setting-up helping pairs where each set member keeps the other in mind and contacts them regularly.

➤ Arranging an informal lunchtime meeting, half-way between regular set meetings.

➤ Encouraging each set member to identify two or three actions that they will take before the next set meeting.

It will also be important for the facilitator to ask the set members for their suggestions – as this will develop their sense of ownership and encourage further creative ideas.

> 'No-one knows what he can do until he tries.'
>
> Publilius Syrus, 442 BC

REFERENCE

1. Kolb D. *Experiential Learning.* Englewood Cliffs, NJ: Prentice-Hall; 1984.

CHAPTER 9

Supporting, recording, ending

SUPPORTING THE ACTION LEARNING PROCESS

There exists a range of support material which can be used as part of the action learning process. This material should, however, be used with care, for it may confuse ends with means – the problem of the tail wagging the dog! However, support material can be helpful because of the innate and overwhelming seductiveness of the particular issue being addressed by the set member, which can lead to them becoming obsessed with action, at the expense of learning. Support material can, therefore, divert people away from this task-obsession and towards learning about the processes by which the task is achieved – and so emphasise the importance of learning, alongside task achievement. Support material forces explicit discussion within the set of the learning processes and achievements within the workplace ('out there') and within the set ('in here').

Such material should only be used when:
➤ It has been presented and described to the set members by the facilitator.
➤ Set members have had sufficient time and opportunity to consider the advantages and disadvantages of using such material.
➤ Individual set members, and the set as a whole, make a conscious decision to use the material.

Support material falls under three main heading – diagnostics, reflection on practice and action planning.

Diagnostics

'The real voyage of discovery consists not in seeking new lands, but with seeing with new eyes.'

Marcel Proust

This is support material which can help set members diagnose the learning and development climate in their organisations and consider the influence of their personal learning styles. Chapter 4 of this book highlighted three tools which can help with such diagnosis.

In addition to these instruments, a number of other questionnaires also exist to help set members assess their own personal learning style. The original work in this field was undertaken by David Kolb[1], as explained in Chapter 3, and his ideas, especially on learning and problem-solving, clearly underlie action learning. The self-diagnostic method which he created – the Learning Style Inventory (LSI) – has, however, been criticised for being culture-bound and has found less favour as time has elapsed. *The Learning Style Questionnaire (LSQ)* devised by Peter Honey and Alan Mumford[2] has proved much more popular. It identifies four learning styles:

Activist: Someone who thrives on learning from challenges and new experiences.

Reflector: Someone who tends to be cautious, standing-back and observing experiences from different perspectives.

Theorist: Someone who adapts and integrates observations into logically sound theories.

Pragmatist: Someone who likes to try-out new ideas, theories and techniques to see whether they work in practice.

Honey and Mumford suggest that everyone develops their own characteristic profile across these four styles, although they also point out that:

➤ A person's learning style is not fixed and is capable of change. Indeed, it does frequently change in response to a variety of external situations and influences.

➤ The information which people gain from the LSQ results should not be used to avoid particular types of learning, but rather should provide a basis for developing an approach to personal learning which results in a more balanced profile.

An action learning set is usually most valuable to individuals when different learning styles are represented within the set membership – and least successful where the individual set members all have the same or similar learning styles. This is the case, despite the mixture of learning styles often causing discomfort to set members. People with different preferences in learning style, and from different areas of experience, often make the best set members precisely because their line of thought provokes the most challenging and enlightening questions from each other.

There is a danger, however, of using the LSQ or other similar assessment tools as a typology – dividing people into discrete categories. When people pin labels on themselves (*'I'm a Pragmatist'*) they might well believe that, once they have identified their predominant learning style, it is a fixed personality trait which cannot be changed, so they must always work within that limitation, seeking only experiences which 'match' their preferred style and hence avoid those that offer a different approach. This could also potentially be reinforced by facilitators, who might foster the idea that people are only really capable of learning in one particular way.

Such a viewpoint is not what Honey and Mumford intended and runs counter to the understandings about adult learning which underpin action learning (*see* Chapter 1). Used with care and sensitivity, the LSQ and other diagnostics can support action learning – with the powerful rider that they must never be mistaken for ends – they are only means to help and stimulate the learning process.

Details about how to access the LSQ are provided in Part 3 of this book.

Reflection on practice

In the sphere of professional clinical practice (doctors, nurses, allied health professionals and others) and its' development, the idea that practice can be improved by structured reflection is a common one,[3] although less well-developed in the managerial sphere, although even here ideas are changing.[4] Three useful approaches which can help set members reflect on what they do are critical incident analysis, learning diaries and biography work. All are based on the reflective cycle model shown in Figure 19.

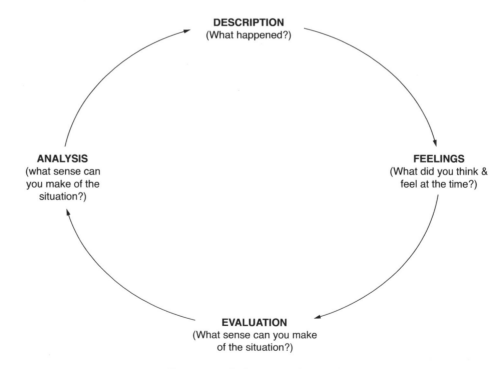

DESCRIPTION
(What happened?)

FEELINGS
(What did you think &
feel at the time?)

EVALUATION
(What sense can you make
of the situation?)

ANALYSIS
(what sense can
you make of the
situation?)

Figure 19: Reflective cycle model

1. *Critical Incident Analysis*: This is an approach which is used to tease out of what people do those aspects which are critical to success or failure, and to find out what behaviours are thus critical to good or poor performance. The emphasis is on the process – with *how* people behave in successful or unsuccessful ways. It typically involves a number of stages:

➤ Describing a significant and recent incident which did or did not meet an intended goal, or in which the individual felt that they were particularly effective or ineffective. The more vivid the description of the incident, the better. Effectively it is a narrative account or story (in chronological order) of the events and processes of the situation – what happened, what the person felt, thought and did.

➤ Reviewing what the person actually did that was effective or ineffective. This might involve:
   - Asking what else might have happened, or what else should have happened.
   - Trying to see what happened from another viewpoint.
   - Asking what did not happen – and why.
   - Considering what really was the cause of the problem.
   - Considering what might have been left out of the narrative.
   - Asking what personal values, beliefs and assumptions underlie the situation.
   - Asking what were the choices in the situation and why particular choices were made.
   - Asking what might be learned from the situation.
   - The processes used in Critical Incident Analysis clearly resonate with the processes of action learning and there are two possible ways in which the former can be used to support the latter. It might, for example, form the basis of the progress-reporting element of set meetings, with a set member offering their narrative and the other set members addressing the questions mentioned above. Alternatively, individual set members might use it privately to prepare for a set meeting – for the questions it poses could provide a useful checklist and enrich the account of their work on the particular issue.

2. *Learning Diaries*: The purpose of a learning diary is twofold – to record the experience of a set member across the duration of the set meetings and to make linkages between what happens in the set and what happens in the workplace – in order to encourage and develop reflection on experience and learning.

➤ As with the use of diagnostics, set members should decide individually and collectively whether the use of a learning diary would be a helpful thing. It is paradoxical that the set members who might benefit most from the reflection which keeping a learning diary stimulates are often those who are most likely to resist adopting this approach! If a learning diary is to be kept then set members will need to:

- Be frank and sincere in what they write.
- Use a variety of means (cartoons, newspaper clippings, quotable quotes, etc.) to aid the reflective process.
- Exercise a degree of self-discipline in order to find the time and space to write-up the learning diary on a regular basis.

➤ To encourage learning the diary will need to be both sequential and reflective. The *sequential* element involves jotting-down notes on a continuing and regular basis under such headings as:

- *People* – the behaviour of those in the set or work situation that make an impact on the set member.
- *Events* – key incidents that take place at work or in the set meeting.
- *Reactions* – what the set member thought, felt, wanted and did.

➤ The *reflective* element involves consideration of:

- *Insights* – Ideas or thoughts that made a significant impact on the set member – either their own conclusions or those of other set members.
- *Learning* – the sense that the set member makes of what's happening to them and others.

➤ Reflective learning can be stimulated by such questions as:

- When did I feel most engaged?
- When did I feel most distanced?
- When did I feel most puzzled?
- When did I feel most affirmed?
- What gaps in my learning did I discover and how should I go about filling them?

➤ In this way, the learning diary should seek to be both retrospective (looking backwards and aiming to understand what has happened) and prospective (looking forward and aiming to decide what to do next).

Review of learning diaries can provide set members with material to bring to the set meeting and there could also be a role for them in the evaluation of action learning programmes (see Chapter 12).

3. *Biography Work*: The scope of action learning extends wider than a single job, problem or organisation. Part of its' concern, is with how individuals make sense of the situations they find themselves in. This means that the focus may extend to the set member's career path and choices – indeed their entire life-cycle, as making personal choices is not confined to occupational or organisational matters, but is shaped by a whole range of diverse influences.

➤ What is loosely called 'biography work' can therefore also be a potential support to set members' learning processes because it offers a means for

people to review their existence in ways that transcend the narrow and a –
historical 'snapshots' that many more analytical approaches embody. It is
an enriched perspective that brings together the past and possible futures
with the present for the purposes of understanding and action and has
been used in action learning to support people seeking to place job and
career choices in a life context.

Two examples of biography-related material – the *Life Goals Exercise* and the
Core Process Exercise are provided in Part 3 of this book.

Biography approaches are highly meaningful for people who are in mid-
career, who are considering a career or life change or who have seldom been
introspective with regard to their own lifestyle and career pattern. Once again,
it should be entirely voluntary whether set members opt to do biography work,
and the earlier caveats about means and ends apply here too.

> 'Life is lived forward, but understood backward.'
>
> Soren Keirkegaard

Action Planning: If the work of action learning sets is to be more than navel
contemplation then effective linkage to the work setting is necessary. At each
set meeting set members should be deciding what action they will be taking
next as a result of the process of dialogue and reflection. Some of those actions
will be short-term, while others will be longer-term, but set members will need
to identify what exactly they intend to do.

An action plan is simply a list of major and minor things which must be
done in order to move from where things are now to a desirable future state, so
an effective plan will focus on that desired future state; be realistic and achiev-
able; be specific, with clearly-defined activities; be time-sequenced, with activities in order and be adaptable.

A good action plan will provide answers to the questions:

➤ *What* needs to happen?
➤ *When* does it need to happen by?
➤ *Who* needs to make it happen?

> 'To put your ideas into action is the most difficult thing in the world.'
>
> Goethe

RECORDING

While what happens in action learning sets is not what happens in a formal
and structured meeting where minutes or notes capture the issues covered and
the decisions made, there can be real value in keeping a record of what goes on

in the set meeting. There can be merit in asking at each set meeting for one person to take responsibility for taking brief notes, copying and circulating them, especially on agreed actions and on requests for specific resources or information. Alternatively, Figure 20 offers a template for recording what goes on in an action learning set meeting.

DATE OF MEETING	
VENUE	
PRESENT	
APOLOGIES	
ISSUES DISCUSSED	
OUTCOMES	
MATTERS TO FOLLOW UP	
WHAT?	
HOW?	
BY WHEN?	
BY WHOM?	
DATE OF NEXT MEETING	
TIME OF NEXT MEETING	
VENUE OF NEXT MEETING	

Figure 20: Recording an action learning set meeting

Individual set members will also want to record what the set meeting meant to them and the *Set Meeting Review Worksheet* in Part 3 of this book provides a means of doing so. Application of this resource is covered in more detail in the chapter on evaluation of action learning.

ENDING

While most action learning sets are created for an agreed and finite time-period, there is often a strong desire on the part of set members for the life of the set to continue. This may be because, for some set members, the combination of support and challenge which they receive from colleagues is fairly unique in relation to the rest of their work or life experience. Yet action learning sets are not permanent entities and the set members and the issues which they address will change over time, so the question of the 'shelf-life' of sets is important.

Given the level of commitment required of set members, any set will need to review regularly whether it is continuing to meet individual needs and there will inevitably come a time when that particular configuration of people and issues is no longer effective for each member. Sets which continue to meet, either out of habit or because it is comfortable to do so, will not be productive.

So ending the life of the set should not be seen as a failure – instead it is a good test of action learning itself if the set knows when to stop, rather than continuing on in a sterile manner. If the set has been working well it will be mature enough to realise that as much has been achieved as can be achieved and that the time has come to stop. The ending of the set is thus part of the development process – a symbol of growth rather than loss.

The final session of a set might well include the following four activities, which the facilitator may initiate:

➤ Set members personally recapturing the way they felt when first coming to the set.
➤ Reflection on the aims and outcomes of the set by discovering what each set member has achieved since the set commenced, and hence a reminder of how far everyone has come.
➤ Reflection on the experience of being in the set by remembering how it had been along the way.
➤ Set members sharing with each other and the facilitator how they are now feeling at the end of the set's life, and saying their goodbyes before moving on.

Ultimately, though, the facilitator must put their faith in the set members saying goodbye as they see fit. Some sets do this in a flood of emotion, while others simply retire to the pub with very little fuss! Some sets agree to continue to meet, but socially rather than for former purposes. Others continue as 'virtual' sets, meeting irregularly, but using e-mail for a continuing dialogue.

The processes which set members have gone through and the relationships which they have built, fostered and maintained will prove valuable to them after the set has ended, in a variety of settings. The lessons learned by set members will continue long after the set itself has gone.

'Ubuntu – I am because we are.'

African proverb

REFERENCES

1. Kolb D. *Experiential Learning*. Englewood Cliffs, NJ: Prentice-Hall; 1984.
2. Honey P, Mumford A. *Using Your Learning Styles*, 2nd ed. Maidenhead: Peter Honey Publications; 1995.
3. Edmonstone J, Mackenzie H. Practice development and action learning. *Pract Dev Health*. 2005; 4(1); 24–32.
4. Vaill P. *Learning as a Way of Being: strategies for survival in a world of permanent white water*. San Francisco, CA: Jossey-Bass; 1996.

CHAPTER 10

Dealing with anxiety in action learning

'There are costs and risks to a programme of action, but they are far less than the long-range risks and costs of comfortable inaction.'

John F. Kennedy

The success of action learning sets can be put at risk by such activity or inactivity as:

➤ Set members not attending set meetings or not following-through on commitments to action they have given at those meetings.
➤ Passive attendance – being there in body but not in mind, or feelings. Not listening or responding to what is said by others.
➤ Set members not preparing for set meetings – just turning-up and expecting 'something' to happen – with the onus of responsibility for that 'something' being on other set members and/or the facilitator.
➤ Set members not having a 'real-time' and relevant issue to discuss.
➤ Yarn-spinning, and using-up time.
➤ Theorising – shifting the focus from the issue itself to theories and concepts about the issue.
➤ Game-playing and undermining others' serious commitment.
➤ Hogging the spotlight and dominating the agenda.
➤ Gossiping – wasting time and avoiding addressing the real issue.

Why does this go on? Probably because what happens in meetings of action learning sets is not solely a rational or intellectual process. Each set member will, in the past, have had both positive and negative learning experiences which they will view through the template of their own emotional and psychological history. These experiences will have also been shaped through membership of work, family and social groupings, and conditioned by broader economic, social and political forces in operation, inside work organisations, and in the larger society. In attempting to bring about change, the psychological factors 'inside' set members interact with their actions in the wider group, organisational and social setting.

Action learning always involves anxiety – as does any real learning. Anxiety is an integral part of being a set member (or a set facilitator). Anxiety contributes to both the success and failure of action learning sets. Set members may feel paralysed by anxiety over how they will be viewed or judged if they engage openly and from their feelings, derived from fear and avoidance. Such anxiety can have destructive or self-limiting effects. However, anxiety can also provide the energy needed to risk being honest, direct, challenging and different – and so can help to shape and inform set members' authority and involvement in set meetings, in addition to the insights and self-insight which they generate. Anxieties within the set, can reinforce the facilitator's feelings of incompetence or reticence with engaging in the complex human dynamics of the group.[1]

Inevitably, therefore, some set members (in common with other adult learners) will face the issue of their anxiety as members of the set – doubts over their ability to cope and low levels of self-esteem. This is so because sets work with the feelings and not just the content of an individual's learning and this can manifest itself in a variety of ways:

➤ **Fear of failure** – in the eyes of the other set members and the facilitator – the latter being perceived as an 'authority figure'. Such people will experience difficulty in taking even calculated risks, will undervalue the importance of feelings, and are seldom spontaneous in their interactions with others.

➤ **Reluctance to join in** – an unwillingness to be playful and creative, with behaviour and ideas, due to a fear of appearing foolish. A reluctance to ask *'What if…?'* resulting in highly 'serious' behaviour.

➤ **A narrow self-view** – a low self-assessment of personal abilities and resources and a resulting 'resource myopia', with an inability or unwillingness to recognise the contribution they might make to helping others address their problems.

➤ **Fear of ambiguity** – an avoidance of matters which lack clarity or where outcomes are unknown or unpredictable. A reluctance to try something out, to see whether it works or not and, an over-emphasis on the known at the expense of the unknown.

➤ **Fear of disorder** – a dislike of complexity (typically labelled as 'confusion') and a preference for order, structure, balance, etc., – often expressed in terms of opposites (right/wrong, good/bad) with a corresponding failure to appreciate and integrate the best from seemingly polarised viewpoints.

➤ **Fear of influencing others** – a concern not to appear as aggressive or 'pushy' and thus a hesitation in identifying with emerging points of view.

Action learning involves working on a problem, asking a difficult question or addressing a contentious issue – and will, therefore, entail a degree of risk (of failure, but also of success). Risk can be generated, for example, by:

➤ People relinquishing earlier roles, ideas and practices.
➤ People creating, finding or discovering, new, more adaptable and feasible ideas, and ways of thinking and acting.
➤ People coping with the instability of changing conditions and, the insecurity which this change provokes.

Risk, in turn, raises these feelings of anxiety and results in the tendency for many people, especially in work settings, to seek sanctuary in the views of experts – who provide anxiety-reducing answers and so offer what can seem like safety and security. By contrast, action learning concentrates on helping people own and focus on *their* problem – with all the messiness, confusion and uncertainty which that entails – rather than relying on expert advice. It encourages people to balance and optimise the paradoxes facing them in groups and organisations, to experiment and develop their *own* solutions, rather than appropriating someone else's, and it emphasises the set member learning how to learn, through the use of the set as a facilitating structure or holding framework, where people can express their worries, hopes and fears. It provides the necessary time and space that people need to reflect, review, develop understanding and plan ahead. The minimal structure provided by the set (chiefly through the establishment of agreed ground-rules) provides a means of containing peoples' anxiety. This is shown in Figure 21.

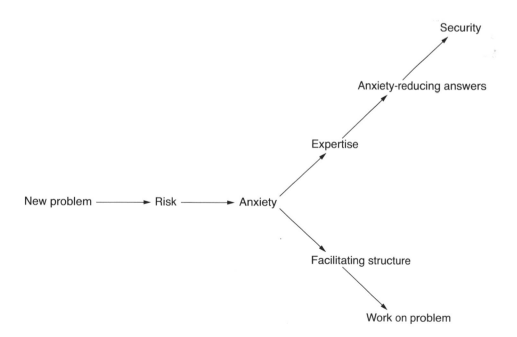

Figure 21: Alternative means of dealing with anxiety

Potentially, the sources of anxiety can include the set member's work role; the particular nature of the problem, issue or question they bring to the set; uncertainty over the purpose and nature of the set itself, and of the set member's place within it. Such anxiety in set members can lead to 'avoidance behaviours'[2] or 'defensive routines',[3] including:

➤ Using the set as a *therapy group,* to explore personal issues at the expense of addressing work-related problems.

➤ The set members acting as a *collective agony aunt* in an advice-giving mode, with little attempt to listen actively to what the set member is saying (and avoiding saying).

➤ Using the set as a *'vicar's tea-party'* or pleasant social gathering – a holiday from the rigours of organisational life.

➤ Set members portraying themselves to other set members as *heroes* (self-idealising) or *villains* (self-deprecating).

It is possible to observe in the operation of action learning sets the phenomenon of 'parallel processing' – dysfunctional behaviour or phenomena reported as being manifest in an organisational setting, also being visible in the working of the set. If this does exist, there is an onus on the set members, and the facilitator, to identify and name the (in-set) behaviour, link it to the reported organisational context and encourage the set member concerned to address it. If the individual set member and/or the other set members are unwilling to do so, there may be a real risk that the set may collapse.

The issue of anxiety is particularly true of action learning in personal service contexts. The idea that the clinical environment, for example, can be a barrier to the implementation of evidence-based research and to developing reflective practice has a long and distinguished pedigree. Revans himself, in a major 1960s study,[4] saw the hospital as an 'institution cradled in anxiety' and the existence of defence mechanisms used by clinical professionals to cope with that anxiety have also been well-documented.[5] More recently, the 'busy-ness' of nurses as a barrier to learning has been emphasised.[6,7.]

Yet the value of the action learning set is that it provides a holding and enabling framework – a transitional space – in which set members' anxiety can be faced, comprehended and worked-through with the appropriate balance of support and challenge from the other set members and the facilitator. They can help to build the confidence of what Revans called their 'comrades in adversity' through empathising with each set member's emotional state at the time they are describing their issue or problem; by seeking to develop increasing levels of respect and trust within the set; by modelling appropriate behaviour to each other, and by addressing such matters directly, rather than indirectly and implicitly. It clearly takes time, but can be done.

'The range of what we think and do is limited by what we fail to notice, and because we fail to notice that we fail to notice, there is little we can do to change, until we notice how failing to notice shapes our thoughts and deeds.'

Ronald Laing

REFERENCES

1. Salecl R. *On Anxiety*. London: Routledge; 2004.
2. Linklater J, Kellner K. Don't just do something...stand there: using action learning to help organisations work with anxiety. *Action Learn Res Pract.* 2008; **5**(2): 167–72.
3. Argyris C. *Overcoming Organisational Defences*. Upper Saddle River, NJ: Prentice-Hall; 1990.
4. Revans R. *Standard For Morale: cause and effect in hospitals*. Oxford: Oxford University Press; 1964.
5. Menzies-Lyth I. *The Functioning of Social Systems as a Defence against Anxiety*. London: Free Association Books; 1970.
6. Wright S, Dolan M. Coming down from the ivory tower. *Prof Nurse*. 1991; **October**: 38–41.
7. Walsh M. How nurses perceive barriers to research implementation. *Nurs Stand*. 1997; **11**(29): 34–9.

CHAPTER 11

Facilitating action learning sets

'Double vision does not require us to stop and think, but the capacity to keep alive, in the midst of action, a multiplicity of views of a situation.'

Donald Schon

Most sets have, or begin life with, a facilitator who is there to enable the learning process to take place, by helping to create conditions which make it possible for set members to learn from their own experience and from that of others. The facilitator is not there to lead the set, or to chair it, or control it. He or she is the *'guide on the side'* rather than the *'sage on the stage'*. Inevitably, the facilitator will be most active in the early life of the set, setting it up, helping set members to find their feet, get to know each other, agree ground-rules, devise a way of working, etc., – to generally 'jump-start' the set (without excessive P!). Thereafter, the facilitator's interventions need to be:

➤ Limited – to when real help can be given.

➤ Judicious – wise and careful.

➤ Tentative – and gentle.

➤ Timely

and, above all

➤ Based on an intention to be helpful and to foster learning.

READING AND NUDGING

The facilitator of action learning sets undertakes two important activities – reading and nudging.[1]

Reading involves recognising the patterns of interaction, activity and interdependence between members of the set – the informal sub-groupings and alliances, the shared experiences and understandings and the differences and tensions. It involves three elements:

➤ *Taking in from the self:* The recognition, and awareness, of what feelings the facilitator is experiencing, and what their reactions to those feelings might be.

➤ *Taking in from the set:* The facilitator listens, watches and senses what is happening in the set at the level of process – with *'how'* people are saying things to each other.

➤ *Making sense of it:* Seeking to distinguish between immediate and short-term matters within the set and longer-term aspects; assessing what behaviour might be unintended and accidental, rather than deliberate, etc. The facilitator does not interpret the set members' behaviour, but simply describes the patterns observed and asks questions based on this.

Nudging involves the facilitator's interventions in the life of the set. Such interventions need to be rare, appropriate and designed to foster the learning either of a single set member or the entire set membership. The facilitator can achieve this by:

➤ Acting as a *role model* for behaviour, which is appropriate to all set members.

➤ Encouraging the *involvement* and *participation* of all set members, especially quieter ones.

➤ *Policing the boundaries* – ensuring that the setting for set meetings is not subject to external interruptions and managing time within the set meetings (adherence to agreed starting and stopping times, equal airtime for all set members).

➤ *Enabling learning* – typically through questions aimed at raising set members' awareness and encouraging their ownership of, and reflection on, the issues which confront them.

In doing so, the facilitator fosters a sense of collective identity among the set members and emphasises their mutual interdependence.

QUALITIES REQUIRED BY FACILITATORS

It is possible to specify the personal qualities that a facilitator needs to display.[2,3] They include:

➤ *Tolerance of ambiguity:* The facilitator operates in a realm of uncertainty and must be prepared to let set members take control from them – unless the facilitator accepts and welcomes this, they will not enjoy the role or undertake it well.

➤ *Openness and frankness:* An ability to recognise and express personal feelings as they arise in the course of a set meeting.

➤ *Patience:* In endless quantities!

➤ *An overwhelming desire to see people learn:* The learning of set members is likely to happen slowly, incrementally, personally and often, privately. So powerful can be the desire to speed things up, that the facilitator

will inevitably spend some of their time 'biting their tongue' and not intervening for fear of upsetting the learning process in the set.
➤ *Empathy:* A sense of standing in another's shoes.
➤ *Understanding the micro-politics of the organisation* – realising how things get done, where power lies and how it might be mobilised for change.
➤ An ability to summarise and portray the 'big picture': Pulling all the strands together to make sense of what is happening, combined with an awareness of the broader context within which the life and work of the set and its' members takes place.
➤ *Self-doubt:* The ability to question the self, to admit personal uncertainties and mistakes in a way that does not threaten the security of the set, but reveals that the facilitator is human too.

There are also qualities which are not needed and can impede the learning of set members. They include:
➤ *'Trainer' skills*: It is no longer necessary to structure the sequencing of sessions and materials as the 'curriculum' is brought by the set members.
➤ *Presentation skills:* The more effective the facilitator is at these skills, the more likely set members may see the facilitator as an expert, and the less likely they will be to continue to lead their own development.
➤ *Fluency:* The use of language in an oratorical sense will detract from the facilitator's need to express what is being seen and felt in an authentic fashion.

Facilitator skills

The skills which an action learning set facilitator needs to develop include:
➤ *Timing of interventions:* Too early and the issue is not understood. Too late and an opportunity for learning may be lost.
➤ *Asking good questions:* These are questions which make set members think and feel, but at the same time feel both supported and challenged, rather than criticised.
➤ *Calibrating action and learning:* If the bulk of the set members' talk is about what they have learned, then the facilitator may need to ask *'What are you going to do?'.* If the bulk of the talk is about action, then the facilitator may need to ask *'What is this saying to you?'.*
➤ *Using the right language*: Different professional and occupational tribes have different languages (jargon, abbreviations, etc.). For example, in medicine the term 'ALS' stands for Advanced Life Support, rather than action learning set! However, the rule for the facilitator is 'only connect' so they need to beware of potential mystification, of talking-down or the seduction of intellectualising.

➤ *Choosing issues that help:* Out of everything which might be going on at any one time within the set, the facilitator chooses those matters that link what's happening in the set with the parallel difficulties that set members may be having back in their organisations.

➤ *Saying nothing and being invisible:* Realising that to intervene at crucial points may interrupt or short-circuit the learning process of an individual set member or the set as a whole.

➤ *Parallel-processing:* The ability to track a number of processes which are taking place in the set at the same time – for most of the time.

➤ *Truthful help:* Making statements truthfully, while structuring the statements to be of maximum benefit, to individual set members or the entire set.

Facilitator development

The role of the action learning set facilitator is founded as much upon adherence to certain personal values, as it is to specific knowledge and skill. It is probably the intention and belief in the importance of the learning process which is the crucial requirement. Facilitators have to believe in the approaches and methods they adopt, based upon their own experience, reflection and dialogue with others.

Facilitating action learning sets does require high-level facilitation skills, but it is possible to learn these skills and techniques, so most people with moderately well-developed interpersonal skills can learn to be an action learning set facilitator.

Those seeking to become action learning set facilitators, or those concerned with developing them, will be aiming to develop:

➤ *Self-insight and understanding* on the part of the facilitator.

➤ Experience of being in, and working with, *a variety of groups* – and consciously learning from the experience of doing so.

➤ An understanding of some *helpful theoretical models*, largely informed by psychology (group processes, roles, norms, stages of group development, etc.), but not specifically, for example, from psychotherapy. Action learning assumes health and growth among set members, rather than illness and instability. Understanding drawn from the arts (literature, poetry, etc.) can be just as useful as that derived from the social or behavioural sciences.

Ultimately, though, it is only by facilitating an action learning set and reflecting on the experience (ideally in concert with others doing the same) that a would-be facilitator can learn how to do it, what it really feels like and whether the experience is a positive one. The implications of this are that:

➤ Future facilitators can be drawn from the ranks of participants in earlier action learning sets, because the insights drawn from being a set member can be extremely useful in developing within the facilitator role.

➤ Structured facilitator development, as well as fostering an understanding of relevant theoretical models and frameworks, should also provide opportunities for practice in the facilitation of groups, for feedback on performance in doing so and for reflection and dialogue on this.

➤ Using the set approach itself can produce the best results. The creation of a set made up of facilitators whose issues relate to the application of action learning in their own organisation, working on an agreed basis with their own facilitator, can effectively use action learning to develop action learning.

Pitfalls for facilitators

Action learning presents a great opportunity for lively and engaged learning, but there can be pitfalls which facilitators need to be aware of. Some of these relate to the operation of the set itself, while others relate to the facilitator's behaviour.

With regard to the *set itself*, the most common pitfall is for the focus on action and learning to be lost. As a meeting of like-minds, an obvious function of the set is a social one – to meet with colleagues and friends, to share highs and lows, achievements and anxieties and to generally 'touch base'. There is real value in all of these things, but it is important not to lose sight of the full range of learning opportunities offered by the set. Some of the dangers include:

➤ *Some set members have been 'volunteered' or sent* – they have not themselves decided to be part of a set and believe, consciously or unconsciously, that they have been sent for remedial purposes. The facilitator, if they are aware of such background, might discuss this personally with the set member, seeking to identify whether set membership is appropriate or not.

➤ *Some set members don't pull their weight and leave it to others to do all the work:* Such a problem needs to be dealt with earlier, rather than later. The longer it is left, the more damage will be done to the set and its' members will become resentful. The issue may need to be placed on the agenda of a set meeting and be addressed directly, based on how set members feel about it. Such a discussion needs to be conducted in positive terms, asking what can be done to ensure that everyone has the chance to contribute.

➤ *The set spends too much time working out what people should be doing, rather than discussing issues and learning from each other's experiences:* This can be tackled early by devoting time at the first meeting of the set so that everyone understands the requisite way of working.

➤ *Set members wander off the point during set meetings and generally have trouble staying focused:* One way of dealing with this can be to have a written agenda or timetable for each set meeting. The facilitator can also check with set members whether they consider that set meetings are going on too long. Enthusiasm and concentration cannot be maintained indefinitely but can be refreshed and maximised by short and frequent breaks (such as coffee, tea and lunch breaks and 'comfort stops' and by regular changes of tack).

In relation to the *facilitator's behaviour*, most pitfalls derive from the facilitator mistaking their own needs for those of the set members. An obvious example would be the tendency for set members to leave it to the facilitator only to notice what is going on and to ask questions, rather than set members taking that responsibility on themselves. Other pitfalls include:

➤ *The temptation of the expert role:* The danger that by falling-back on the expert role, the facilitator encourages passivity among set members – and a false sense of confidence in the facilitator!

➤ *The seduction of rescuing:* This can happen when a facilitator gives in to the urge to rescue a set member who is struggling with a particularly difficult question, and offers them specific suggestions about what they must do to resolve their issue.

➤ *Mistaking the means as the end:* This involves 'padding-out' the work of the set with small and incremental assignments which, over time, change the process of the set meeting into that of a more traditional learning programme. The caveats mentioned in Chapter 8 about the use of support material particularly apply here.

> 'The test of a first-rate intelligence is the ability to hold two opposed ideas in the mind at the same time and still retain the ability to function.'
>
> F. Scott Fitzgerald

REFERENCES

1. Havergal M, Edmonstone J. *The Facilitator's Toolkit.* Aldershot: Gower Publishing; 2003.
2. Casey D. The emerging role of the set adviser in action learning. *J Eur Ind Train.* 5(3): 155–66.
3. Pedler M. *Action Learning For Managers.* London: Lemos & Crane; 1996.

CHAPTER 12

Variations on the action learning theme

Although the norm for action learning appears to be the set working with a facilitator across a period of time, there are also a number of variations on this theme. Three of these are examined here – auto-action learning, virtual action learning sets and self-facilitated action learning.

AUTO-ACTION LEARNING

A recent account[1] explains how the membership of an individual in an action learning set can be supplemented by what they term 'auto-action learning'. Based around the questions posed in the Action Learning Problem Brief (see Table 5, page 52) the use of a mentor outside of the set provided an opportunity for reflection, learning and the devising of planned actions. This appeared to speed-up learning and act as a motivator to apply experience from elsewhere to the problem situation. It also served to build the principle of the empowerment of the problem-holder through using the format (the Action Learning Problem Brief) already established in use within the set.

Auto-action learning therefore seems to involve a series of parallel relationships (set membership and mentoring) which serve to reinforce each other. The use of the structured format focused attention both retrospectively (on learning achieved) and prospectively (on forward action). The authors concluded that the use of such systematic headings helped to keep a focus on motivation, learning and review.

VIRTUAL ACTION LEARNING SETS

Faced with the busy life most professionals and managers lead, the question of whether 'virtual' action learning sets can offer a valid alternative to the face-to-face interaction which ordinary set provide is often raised.[2] Figure 22 shows six potential forms of virtual action learning (VAL):

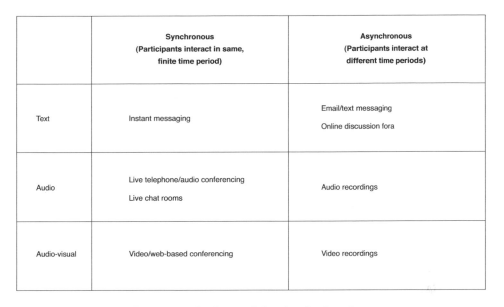

	Synchronous (Participants interact in same, finite time period)	Asynchronous (Participants interact at different time periods)
Text	Instant messaging	Email/text messaging Online discussion fora
Audio	Live telephone/audio conferencing Live chat rooms	Audio recordings
Audio-visual	Video/web-based conferencing	Video recordings

Figure 22: Six forms of virtual action learning

At present, virtual action learning remains experimental and pioneering and highly diverse in its' many manifestations which operate in a diverse range of organisational contexts, and in pursuit of a variety of different objectives. While it appears to work well in certain contexts, and offers great potential for further research and use in different organisational and educational learning contexts, it also raises a number of relevant questions, such as how virtual sets can be facilitated and the nature of virtual group dynamics. Two possible approaches – email and audio-conferencing – are considered here.

E-mail

E-mail potentially offers a single (one-to-one) communication channel between set members, but one that filters-out many of the significant non-verbal clues as to how strongly they may feel about the issue in question – and so represents a fairly impersonal means of communication with reduced language variety. Moreover, communication does not take place in 'real-time' – there is a delay in which set members can (if they so wish) mask strong feelings and manage the impression which they present to their virtual colleagues. E-mail also has a poor image – many people do not reply to e-mails and a communication from another set member which is 'lost' within a backlog of e-mails is unlikely to receive the attention which it deserves, placed as it is, alongside minutes of meetings, diary dates, inquiries, etc.

Audio-conferencing

This approach, using telephone communication in what is termed conference call mode, potentially offers a more positive way forward, although it too is not without its' drawbacks. It is clearly not as powerful as face-to-face set meetings and evidence from use suggests that:

➤ The approach works well with people who are already comfortable with audio-conferencing.

➤ There are advantages in set members knowing each other reasonably well in advance of the set or at least having the first meeting face-to-face before moving to a virtual mode.

➤ Set members need to commit to the session as if they were present physically – devoting their full attention to it. Likely distractions should be minimised for the duration of the session or explained in advance.

➤ Set members need a higher level of listening skills and the ability to sense what the other person is saying without visual clues.

➤ A 'natural' time-limit of 2.5 hours is the most feasible, provided set members have hands-free phones and a break is taken.

➤ People taking part should be in a private area where others cannot hear what is said. Hands-free phones must not be audible outside this private area. Where necessary, doors must be marked to advise people not to interrupt.

➤ Details of conference calling arrangements need to be treated as confidential.

SELF-FACILITATED ACTION LEARNING

The eventual goal of an action learning set facilitator must be to make him- or herself redundant as the set members become more mature and experienced in working together. Ultimately, the services of the facilitator are dispensable, but it is for the set to decide when. Abandoning a set too early or outstaying the welcome are both dangers facilitators face.

The process of exiting the set probably needs to be explicit from the start and the facilitator might say, at a fairly early stage *'We will need to decide at what point my presence will not be needed.'* Note the emphasis on 'we' – it is a joint process. Alternatively, the facilitator might ask the set members to review the facilitator role, and how it is working out, after an agreed number of meetings. If the role becomes less and less necessary, it might become sensible for the facilitator to attend set meeting by invitation only – as and when the set membership feel that it would be necessary and helpful to the learning process of the set – for example, when set members have reached an impasse and feel themselves 'stuck'.

Revans himself saw only a limited role for facilitators at the start-up stage and certainly not on an on-going basis.[3] However, current practice[4] deviates from Revans' 'classical principles' in making use of facilitators across the life of the set. However, self-facilitated or self-managed action learning is championed by the Management Development Research Unit at the University of Brighton.[5] In such an approach:

➤ The term 'facilitator' is replaced by that of 'set manager' and undertaken by set members.

➤ Set meetings are more structured and less free-form. Specifically, there are two rounds of time-slots – one is *retrospective* and focuses on reflection and looking back to help learn the lessons of experience, and the other is *prospective* – looking forward to identify the actions needed to move set members forward.

Self-facilitated sets will be a viable option, particularly where the membership of a set is sufficiently experienced and mature – perhaps from earlier membership of other sets – so that they can operate in a self-facilitating mode. However, to do so demands:

➤ A high personal commitment from all set members to attend and to share the work of facilitation as agreed.

➤ Clear agreement among set members about the format to be followed for set meetings and clarity over the roles to be adopted. For example, will facilitation be undertaken collectively (by all and at any time) or will each set member take it in turn at different set meetings to act as facilitator?

➤ A high degree of honesty in running the review of each set meeting so that the set does not collude, for example, to ignore or avoid discussing unhelpful behaviour.

REFERENCES

1. Learmonth A. Pedler M. Auto action learning: a tool for policy change: building capacity across the developing regional system to improve health in the north east of England. *Health Policy.* 2004; **68**(2): 169–81.

2. Pedler M, Dickenson M, Burgoyne J. Virtual action learning. *People Management.* 2005; **October**: 8.

3. Revans R. *The ABC of Action Learning*, 3rd ed. London: Lemos & Crane; 1998.

4. Pedler M, Burgoyne J, Brook C. What has action learning learned to become? *Action Learn Res Pract.* 2005; **2**(1): 49–68.

5. O'Hara S, Bourner T, Webber T. The practice of self-managed action learning. *Action Learn Res Pract.* 2004; **1**(1): 29–42.

CHAPTER 13

Evaluating action learning

'Faced with the choice between changing one's mind and proving that there is no need to do so, almost everybody gets busy on the proof.'

John Kenneth Galbraith

Benefits are claimed for action learning at both the individual and organisational levels – the former in terms of individual performance and personal development and the latter in terms of developed capacity and capability. Before examining the question of evaluation of action learning, it is important to be clear about what is claimed as individual and organisational benefits.

INDIVIDUAL BENEFITS

At the level of the individual, action learning claims to provide real opportunities for personal growth and learning. Set members face real issues and problems which they own and are committed to make real progress on them. They, therefore, need to reflect on how their actions, personal style, values and motivations make an impact on others. The set's focus on action and review helps individuals to experiment and try out different approaches, thereby enhancing their self-awareness. Specifically, therefore, for the individual it is claimed that action learning can bring about:

➤ Greater breadth of understanding, as a basis for building relationships across an organisation or organisations and taking action.
➤ An improved ability to make sense of ambiguous data and situations and address complex problems.
➤ An enhanced capacity to understand and initiate organisational changes.
➤ An increased focus on what makes a difference in a situation.
➤ People who are more action-focused and proactive in delivering results.
➤ Greater effectiveness in communicating proposals to senior managers and leaders.
➤ An enhanced self-awareness of personal impact on others, contributing to an improved ability to work with others in teams.
➤ A developed flexibility in responding to changing situations and adopting a more diverse range of behaviours.

➤ Shared knowledge and learning from a wide range of colleagues.
➤ Legitimate and protected problem-solving time.
➤ Identification of personal and professional development needs.

ORGANISATIONAL BENEFITS

At the level of the organisation (or organisations) action learning claims that benefits will include:

➤ An integrated path to personal and organisational learning at as fast a rate as changes in the outside world.
➤ Enabling effective action to be taken to resolve difficult problems – to do things differently and to continuously improve.
➤ The encouragement of effective teamwork and inter-departmental, inter-professional and inter-organisational co-operation.
➤ The development of leaders with a flexible and more entrepreneurial approach.
➤ A focusing of the energies of committed people.
➤ A complementary and supporting activity to mentoring, coaching and other work-based development approaches.

PROBLEMS WITH EVALUATION

While everyone can agree on the importance of and need for evaluation of any change process or developmental activity, the evidence strongly suggests that such processes and activities continue to follow one after the other, with little evaluation of their impact before organisations progress on to the next. Among the reasons for this are that, in seeking to evaluate developmental activity, it is relatively easy to collect data on *reactions* (thoughts and feelings); slightly more difficult, but not impossible, to collect data on *learning* (knowledge, skills and attitudes gained or changed); more problematic to collect data on changes in performance *behaviour* and very difficult indeed to collect data on *outcomes* (the impact or effect of changed behaviour on organisational performance).[1] The move from reactions to outcomes introduces a significant number of intervening variables (other things going on in the organisation) which make it more difficult (some would say impossible) to ascribe simple cause-and-effect relationships.

Nevertheless, recent evaluation of change activity has been marked by a shift of emphasis from outputs to *outcomes* (the difference that the particular intervention has made) and from purely quantitative to a judicious mix of *quantitative and qualitative* methods. Major issues include:

➤ *Time:* How to evaluate interventions over the short-term that are intended to have longer-term impacts? One possible way forward is 'intermediate measurement' or assessment of distance travelled so far.

➤ *Complexity:* As highlighted above, where there are potentially multiple intervening variables, how can the effects of one programme or activity be disentangled from the others, especially when they may overlap? One response may be to conclude it is not possible to identify causality conclusively, or perhaps only at the micro or individual level.

➤ *Value:* What actually counts as 'success'? What is valued and by whom? Useful responses include including all the key stakeholders in the evaluation process and seeking to 'surface' the assumptions behind programmes and activities – what are people trying to do through them?

➤ *Horses for courses:* The size of the evaluation needs to be in proportion to the programme being evaluated and the form evaluation takes should reflect the values underlying the programme itself.

One alternative suggestion is to rely on the processes of informal evaluation that occur continually at every level of an organisation.[2] Rather than emphasising systematic and planned measurement, it is suggested that the key may lie in focusing on processes that facilitate and encourage dialogue across professional, managerial and organisational boundaries; the pooling of experiences and informal assessment that has the potential to lead to shared learning.

PROBLEMS WITH EVALUATING ACTION LEARNING

Chapter 1 spelled-out that action learning was based on an 'inside-out' development process, rather than an 'outside-in' process. The latter approach tends to see action learning as only a *tool* – an instrumental means of reaching previously-defined ends and an expression of an 'instrumentalist' ethos.[3] It is concerned, to use action learning parlance, with *puzzles* (where there are simple right and wrong answers) and with *single-loop learning* (basic error-detection and correction – *see* Chapter 3). However, action learning deals with *problems* (messy, complex and inter-dependent 'tangles' where *double-loop learning* (challenging and modifying assumptions and practices) is essential.

Moreover, it is difficult, perhaps even impossible, to predict specific outcomes from action learning in advance and in detail. The starting or presenting problem that a set member arrives with may change or evolve from interactions and dialogue with other set members and the facilitator. The set member may experience insight into their own behaviour or the culture of their organisation that stimulates action which was not predictable prior to the set being created. This can include, for example, individuals going on to make career choices (to move into or out of particular roles or organisations) which may be highly positive from the individual's viewpoint, but much less so from that of the organisation! The outcomes of action learning are therefore potentially open-ended and sometimes unpredictable.

There can be seen to be four levels to successful action learning[4] and they are:

➤ *Level 1:* Problem-solving in relation to a specific task or problem.
➤ *Level 2:* Level 1, plus reframing of the problem or issue and a conscious transfer of skill.
➤ *Level 3:* Levels 1 and 2, plus self-insight into personal learning styles and other aspects of personal development.
➤ *Level 4:* Levels 1, 2 and 3, plus a focus on the organisation's culture and on life and career issues.

Thus, claim the authors, the more successful action learning is, the more it moves from Level 1 towards Level 4.

One large-scale impact evaluation of action learning in the NHS[5] concluded that it had made a major impact on many individuals, but little overall impact on the organisations concerned. At the other extreme, as was pointed-out in Chapter 1, the application of a Return On Investment (ROI) approach to action learning across a range of commercial enterprises suggested significant cost-saving achieved and the fostering of revenue-raising initiatives.[6] It will become increasingly important for action learning to show some evidence base for its' efficacy and this means that evaluation must become a normal process associated with action learning programmes.

TWO TYPES OF EVALUATION

There is a need to distinguish between two different types of evaluation. Some evaluation is formative (or developmental). It is concerned with steering and improving action learning while it is happening. Other evaluation is summative (or judgemental) and is concerned with assessing the impact or contribution of action learning. These two evaluation approaches can be presented as 'ideal types' for the purposes of comparison,[7] as shown in Figure 23.

Formative (within-set) evaluation should be part of the on-going work of each action learning set meeting and two activities are provided in the Resources section to assist this process. They are the Set Meeting Review Worksheet and the Support/Challenge Map. Such resources can be used, or on a more informal basis, there can be value in reviewing ground-rules, participants' views on the set process, balance between support and challenge and participants' progress with their issue at about three or four meetings into the set's life. The focus is clearly on evaluating progress with learning and reviewing the helpful and less helpful norms of the set – to make future meetings more productive.

In practice, the evaluation of action learning needs to address both summative and formative issues, as the case study below suggests.

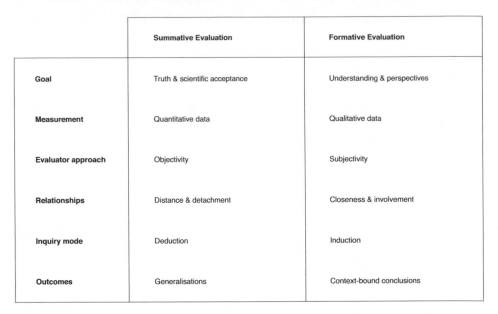

	Summative Evaluation	Formative Evaluation
Goal	Truth & scientific acceptance	Understanding & perspectives
Measurement	Quantitative data	Qualitative data
Evaluator approach	Objectivity	Subjectivity
Relationships	Distance & detachment	Closeness & involvement
Inquiry mode	Deduction	Induction
Outcomes	Generalisations	Context-bound conclusions

Figure 23: Summative and formative evaluation

EVALUATING ACTION LEARNING: A CASE STUDY

During 2003–04, the author and a colleague facilitated action learning sets for people who wanted to develop their skills in setting-up and running sets, within their own organisations. Two sets of six people ran broadly in parallel, the client for the work being the Trent Strategic Health Authority. Funding became available from the National Primary and Care Trust Development Programme (NatPaCT) to support an evaluation, although this initiative arose as the sets were coming to an end. Funding was limited so the evaluation comprised:

➤ **Telephone interviews** with key stakeholders in the two large employing NHS teaching hospital Trusts who had people on the programme to check their motivation in supporting the programme.

➤ A **questionnaire** for all set members administered after the end of the set meetings.

The questionnaire collected some 'biographical' data (gender, age, job background, time in post, attendance) but concentrated on such matters as:

➤ Set members previous experience of action learning.

➤ How set members became aware of the development opportunity afforded by the sets.

➤ Set members' motivation for involvement.

➤ The nature of the presenting problem set members brought to the set and how it evolved throughout the life of the set.

➤ Progress made on the issue or problem and what had been learned from working on it.
➤ Perceptions of how relevant set membership was to personal development needs.
➤ Sustainability – what learning had taken place which would help on a continuing basis.
➤ The impact made on individuals by set membership.
➤ Common themes identifiable across the work of the set.
➤ Appropriateness of facilitator style.
➤ Level at which the set operated (see above). Set members were asked to allocate 100 points across the four levels to illustrate this.
➤ Suggestions for improvement to design and process.
➤ Personal learning achieved.

Data was collected by both closed and open questions, rating scales and the allocation process mentioned above.

The evaluation study revealed that:
➤ There was a high degree of congruence between the rationale of employing organisations and set members with regard to the purpose and intended outcomes.
➤ Set members opted for action learning in response to work-related problems or through self-initiative.
➤ The sets were experienced as highly relevant to set members' development needs, with the facilitators' style being experienced as very appropriate.
➤ Learning achieved was both specific to problems/issues brought or surfaced, but also generic and transferable on a sustainable basis to other situations.
➤ There were important differences between the two sets in terms of gender, age, time in post, level of working.
➤ A number of improvements to the design of future programmes were suggested.

EVALUATING ACTION LEARNING PROGRAMMES: A CHECKLIST

The main challenge in evaluating action learning is to ensure that the evaluation process is fit-for-purpose – in other words, that it is appropriate to the activity or programme being evaluated. The following are some useful questions to consider when planning the evaluation process:
➤ What do we *want to know* about the programme?
➤ Who or what was the programme *for*?
➤ What are the programme's *objectives*? Are they clear?
➤ Who are the key *stakeholders*? What are their *expectations* of the evaluation?

➤ What *benefits* is the evaluation intended to provide? Will the evaluation provide *useful insights* (and to whom)? Will it provide *timely insights*? Will it generate *new insights* and not duplicate other work?

➤ What are the *costs* or resource implications of evaluation – in terms of time and money?

➤ Will the benefits of the evaluation *outweigh* the costs?

➤ *Who is the information for*? Internal? External? Both?

➤ *When/how often* will the information be needed?

➤ In what *form* is the information required?

➤ How should the information be *collected and analysed*? By whom?

➤ Will the evaluation be conducted in a manner that is *acceptable* to the key stakeholders – i.e., with sensitivity?

➤ Will the evaluation contribute to the *evidence-base* of 'what works in what circumstances and why'? Will it move us forward?

Answers to these questions will provide the basis of an evaluation framework for an action learning programme. The framework will also need to meet five criteria:

➤ The evaluation process will need to generate sufficient information to meet the requirement of *accountability* – i.e., that resources have been deployed appropriately.

➤ It will need to provide information that is *useful* to the programme or activity itself and for other existing or planned future programmes – and have clear implications for *action* – not just a 'one the one hand and on the other' conclusion.

➤ The evaluation process will need to be *easy to manage and implement* within the resources available.

➤ The approach chosen needs to be able to stand up to *external scrutiny*, with adequate rigour in both quantitative and qualitative terms.

➤ The process will need to include *dissemination* of findings in an accessible form to the appropriate people – stakeholders and others.

Finally, it is important to remember that, as a recent review of evaluation of leadership development initiatives in the NHS concluded:

> 'Evaluation can only ever provide good quality information to inform decision-making. It is unlikely to supply ready-made answers because the results will need to be interpreted as part of a process of discussion and judgement, with the views of different stakeholders and the intended outcomes of the activity being taken into account'.[8]

> 'In order to arrive at what you do not know, you must go by the way which is the way of ignorance.'
>
> T.S. Eliot

REFERENCES

1. Kirkpatrick D, Kirkpatrick J. *Evaluating Training Programs: the four levels.* 4th ed. San Francisco, CA: Berrett-Koehler; 1998.

2. Skinner D. Evaluation and change management: rhetoric and reality. *Hum Res Manag J.* 2004; **14**(3): 5–19.

3. Furedi F. *Where have all the Intellectuals Gone? confronting twenty-first century philistinism.* London: Continuum Press; 2004.

4. Yorks Y, O'Neil J, Marsick V. Action learning: theoretical bases and varieties of practice. In: Yorks Y, O'Neil J, Marsick V, editors. *Action Learning: successful strategies for individual, team and organisation development.* Baton Rouge: Academy of Human Resource Management; 1999.

5. Weiland G, Leigh H. *Changing Hospitals.* London: Tavistock Publications; 1971.

6. Wills G, Oliver C. Measuring the return on investment from management action learning. *Manag Dev Rev.* 1996; **9**(1): 17–21.

7. Thackwray R, Box M. Organisation development in higher education: evaluation of learning and development. *HESDA Paper.* 2001

8. Larsen L, Cummins J, Brown H, *et al. Learning from Evaluation: summary of reports of evaluations of leadership initiatives.* London: Office for Public Management/NHS Leadership Centre; 2005.

CHAPTER 14

How action learning has evolved

'When the world is predictable you need smart people, but when the world is unpredictable you need adaptable people.'

Henry Mintzberg

GENERAL EVOLUTION

A recent overview[1] surveyed the development of action learning within the UK and charted the evolution from the original concepts developed by Revans. It identifies 'Revans' Classical Principle', a shorthand for the consistencies within the reading of Reg Revans' considerable output (over a period of more than 50 years). Indeed, Revans endorsed many different forms of action learning at different times in his long career and his own concepts evolved over that time. As another commentator has highlighted:

'Reg Revans outlined the principles of action learning – but not always how to implement them. His ideas were never a package of delivery.'[2]

The Classical Principles are said to include:
➤ The requirement for action as the basis for learning.
➤ Profound personal development resulting from reflection upon action.
➤ Working with problems (with no 'right' answers) and not puzzles (susceptible to expert knowledge).
➤ Problems being sponsored and aimed at organisational as well as personal development.
➤ Action learners working in sets of peers ('comrades in adversity') to support and challenge each other.
➤ The search for fresh questions and Q (Questioning Insight) takes primacy over access to expert knowledge (or P).

The research which the article reports concluded that:
➤ Action learning had spread as an *ethos* (or general way of thinking about learning) as well as a *method* (specific set of practices).
➤ Different practices and approaches to action learning were being developed in different locations and communities. While there was widely shared agreement on the ethos, there were wide variations in method or practice.

➤ There had been significant departures or evolutions from the Classical Principles of Revans, which included:

- A shift to individual choice of the problems or issues addressed and away from negotiated agreements with sponsors or commissioners of action learning in the organisation. The issue chosen is likely to relate to 'own job' issues and therefore fall within Cells 1 and 2 of Figure 16 in Chapter 5 (*see* page 63).

- A concomitant focus of action learning on personal development issues with less of a concentration on organisational problems.

- A set size of around 6 people.

- The use of permanent facilitators working with sets throughout their life-cycle. This is something never endorsed by Revans who saw a role only for 'initiators' who helped sets to get started and then left, rather than having a permanent presence.

- The use of action learning in Higher Education as part of (and an adjunct to) qualification programmes which also involve teaching.

- Variations from the Classical Principles as alternatives to action learning 'practice norms' – as outlined in Chapter 11.

- However, the authors highlighted some caveats about their work, noting a lack of response from large private sector businesses and consultancies, so the picture presented might not be completely accurate.

- A further intriguing emergent issue is the extent to which action learning processes are culturally defined. There is a growing literature on cultural differences in relation to interpersonal communication[3,4,5,6] and this suggests that, as a fairly intimate approach to group working, action learning may be more difficult for some groups and individuals. This may operate at the level of country-based cultural differences as well as those of gender. It has been suggested, for example, that women set members are more at ease with disclosure of their personal attitudes and issues than men.[7]) Certainly, action learning set facilitators will need to be sensitive to cultural and sub-cultural differences within sets. However, different sets agree different ground-rules and build different norms in relation to the amount of disclosure they feel comfortable with and this can usually be accommodated within the work of the set.

EVOLUTION OF ACTION LEARNING IN THE NHS

From the outset action learning and the NHS have been intimately interlinked. Indeed, Revans' work at Manchester Royal Infirmary in the early 1960s[8] and later with the Hospital Internal Communication (HIC) project in that same decade[9,10] together with further work in learning disability services in the 1970s[11] suggest that healthcare has been one of the 'proving-grounds' for action learning. From early work with healthcare managers, action learning has also spread into a range of health-related fields, including health promotion,[12] nursing,[13,14] mid-wifery,[15,16,17] nurse education,[18,19] public health,[20,21] mental health,[22,23,24] learning disability[25] and practice development.[26] Most of the applications have been of a 'siloed' uni-professional kind, although there have also been some multi-professional applications in clinical governance,[27] primary care,[28] information technology,[29] knowledge management,[30,31] inter-professional working,[32,33,34] multi-agency working[35] and clinical leadership.[36] The relationship between action learning and healthcare has been described as symbiotic and 'benign'.[37]

A recent review of the use of action learning in the NHS[38] identified three main contexts for action learning in healthcare:

1. Action learning as a planned and timetabled activity interwoven with the other formal aspects of a development programme, with the action learning set either ceasing at the end of the programme or being allowed or encouraged to continue in a self-managed way for as long as set members derive benefits.

Examples of this would include the Royal College of Nursing Clinical Leadership Programme[39] and leadership development programmes for General Practitioners.[40]

2. Action learning as an activity introduced towards the end of a formal programme, with the organiser's anticipation that some participants would form an action learning set as a way of continuing their development, bridging the potential guide between the programme and work.

Examples would include the use of action learning sets as a support mechanism for nurses and allied health professionals following their participation in the Leading an Empowered Organisation (LEO) programmes which formed part of national clinical leadership development for nurses and allied health professionals.[41]

3. Action learning as a discrete leadership development activity in its' own right, neither relying nor continuing the momentum of a formal programme.

There are ample examples of this, including a wide range of programmes sponsored by the former National Primary and Care Trust Development Programme (NatPaCT) – for the Chief Executives and Professional Executive Committee Chairs of Primary Care Trusts, Primary Care Trust Risk Managers, Allied Health Professionals on the Professional Executive Committees of PCTs, etc. The Integrated Care Network has also made use of this approach, which seems to be particularly useful for people in new and emerging roles dealing with novel and leading-edge issues.

ACTION LEARNING IN A WIDER CONTEXT

In the article mentioned above Pedler *et al.* offer a cognitive map indicating where action learning 'fits'. They propose a framework for thinking about the positioning of action learning based on three positions (as shown in Figure 24):

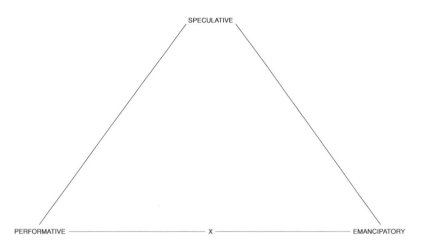

Figure 24: A cognitive map of action learning

1. **Speculative:** This is learning for its own sake, unconcerned with application to practice and concerned with theoretical rigour.
2. **Emancipatory:** This is learning helps to overcome oppression and attain the highest human potential. It is concerned with the holistic development of the person in the world.
3. **Performative:** This is learning that helps action in the world; that resolves problems and produces better services and goods. It is concerned with improving, modernising management and performance.

Pedler *et al.* position action learning at point X between Performative and Emancipatory, commenting that:

> 'Action learning is optimistic, humanistic, engaging, but also pragmatic and sceptical, suspicious of canonical ideas (and the experts who trade in them) and distrustful of speculative knowledge untested in action.'

They also make reference to two 'moral syndromes'[42] of the *Guardian* 'keepers of the sacred flame' of Revans' Classical Principles (anathematising deviations) and the *Trader* (connecting-up different communities of action learning practice, exploring variations, learning from them and modifying own practice). The challenge, they claim is to be *both* Guardians (of the action learning ethos) and Traders (of different methods).

Recent commentators have seen the increasing necessity of developing the ability of learning how to learn for economic, social and political reasons. It has been suggested, [43] using the notion of 'figure and ground' drawn from Gestalt psychology, that achieving immediate learning goals is the 'figure' of any learning activity but the 'ground' is the development of our intuitive understanding of, and expertise at, the learning process itself. As we learn what to do, we also change how we know, and how we come to know.

If what we know about the future is that we do not know much about it, then the key responsibility is not to give people tools that may be out-of-date before they have even been fully mastered, but to help them to become confident and competent designers and makers of their own learning tools as they go along. Another analogy is that people increasingly need to become map-makers and not just readers and interpreters of others' maps.

In all walks of life, new and better ways of doing things can be discovered only if experiment and diversity are permitted. The success of experiments cannot, of course, be guaranteed in advance, so innovators must have some scope of getting things wrong without being punished. This scope is what engineers term 'redundancy' – the capability to deal with unlikely eventualities. Creating redundant capacity means allowing space for diversity and experiment, much of which may be wasted, but without which new eventualities cannot be provided for. The action learning set is just such a potential space.

With its focus on learning how to learn action learning is well-placed to be an increasingly relevant and powerful development approach (both ethos and method(s)) in the 21st century. Moreover, there is an argument to be made that action learning can help to make us good citizens of a democracy. It has been suggested that it:

> 'helps us to take an active stance towards life and helps us overcome the tendency to think, feel and be passive towards the pressures of life.'[44]

> 'We must be the change we wish to see in the world.'

Mahatma Ghandi

REFERENCES

1. Pedler M, Burgoyne J, Btook C. What has action learning learned to become? *Action Learn Res Pract.* 2005; **2**(1): 49–68.
2. Margerison C. Editorial. *Training Journal.* 2000; **November**: 12.
3. Hofstede G, Hofstede G. *Culture and Organisations: software of the mind.* 2nd ed. New York, NY: McGraw-Hill; 2005.
4. Joynt P, Warner M. *Managing Across Cultures.* London: International Thomson Business Press; 1996.
5. Hampden-Turner C, Trompenaars F. *Building Cross-cultural Competence: how to create wealth from conflicting values.* Chichester: Wiley; 2000.
6. Hickson D, Pugh D. *Management Worldwide: distinctive styles amid globalisation.* London: Penguin; 2001.
7. Beaty L. *Action Learning.* York: Learning & Teaching Support Network CPD Paper 1; 2003.
8. Revans R. *Standard for Morale: cause and effect in hospitals.* Oxford: Oxford University Press; 1964.
9. Weiland G, Leigh H. *Changing Hospitals.* London: Tavistock Publications; 1971.
10. Revans R. *Hospitals: communication, choice and change: the hospital internal communications project seen from within.* London: Tavistock Publications; 1972.

11. Collin A, Sturt J. *Report of an Evaluation Study of an Action Learning Project in Hospitals for the Mentally Handicapped, North Derbyshire Health District.* Sheffield: Trent Regional Health Authority, Organisation Development Unit; 1976.

12. Beattie A. Action learning for health on campus. In: Tsouros A, Dowding G, Thompson J, Dooris M, editors. *Health Promoting Universities.* Copenhagen: World Health Organization (Europe); 1998.

13. O'Connell C. *First Steps: the development of an inquiry culture in an acute hospital using action learning.* London: Florence Nightingale Foundation; 2002.

14. Wilson V, Walsh R, Ho A. Using action research and action learning to support and facilitate a change in nursing handover. *J Clin Nurs.* 2006; 3: 35–42.

15. Brownlee M, Foy R. Evidence-based midwifery care: evaluation of a pilot action learning programme. *Practice Midwife.* 2000; 3: 23–6

16. Rogan K. The introduction of action learning into a midwifery curriculum. *Paper presented at Bournemouth University conference, Collaboration in health & social care*; 2003.

17. Mead M, Yearley C, Lawrence C, *et al.* Action learning: a learning and teaching method in the preparation programme for supervisors of midwives. *Action Learn Res Pract.* 2006; 3(2): 175–86.

18. Haddock J. Reflection in groups: contextual and theoretical considerations within nurse education and practice. *Nurs Educ Today.* 1997; 17: 381–5.

19. Jones K, Bunker J, Heywood S, *et al.* Action learning to provide continuing professional development. *Nurse Prescribing.* 2005; 3: 156–8.

20. Carlson C, Wright J. *Enabling the Development of Public Health Networks: national public health network action learning set programme summary report.* Oxford: Public Health Resource Unit & Department of Health; 2004.

21. Learmonth A. Action learning as a tool for developing networks and building evidence-based practice in public health. *Action Learn Res Pract.* 2005; 2(1): 97–104.

22. Spurrell M. Consultant learning groups in psychiatry: report on a pilot study. *Psychiatr Bull.* 2000: 24; 390–2.

23. Onyett S. Leadership for change in mental health services. *Ment Health Rev.* 2002; 7: 20–23.

24. West P. Blackburn with Darwen action learning set: a model for improving the interface between inpatient and community teams. *Ment Health Rev.* 2005.

25. Sutton D. *Action Learning in Hospitals for the Mentally Handicapped.* Southport: Action Learning Projects International Ltd; 1977.

26. Edmonstone J, Mackenzie H. Practice development and action learning. *Pract Dev Health.* 2005; 4(1): 24–32.

27. Boston D, Carter M. Action learning for clinical governance. *Organisations and People.* 2002; 9: 22–7.

28. Emerson T, Morley V, Bell C. ALS support for GP projects. *Organisations and People.* 1999; 6: 17–23.

29. Findlay P, Marples C. Experience in using action learning sets to enhance information management and technology strategic thinking in the UK National Health Service. *J Manag Stud.* 1998; **7**: 165–83.

30. Giles G. Report on accreditation action learning sets in the West Midlands region of the NHS. *Health Libr Rev.* 2000; **17**: 18–188.

31. Booth A, Sutton A, Falzon L. Working together: supporting projects through action learning. *Health Information and Libraries Journal.* 2003; **20**: 225–31.

32. Curtis-Jenkins G, White J. Action learning: a tool to improve inter-professional collaboration and promote change. *J Interprof Care.* 1994; **8**: 265–73.

33. Foy R, Tidy N, Hollis S. Inter-professional learning in primary care: lessons from an action learning programme. *Br J Clin Govern.* 2002; **7**: 40–4.

34. Wilson D, Jones H. Working with GPs and hospital consultants in developing clinical leadership in a health community. In: Edmonstone J, editor. *Clinical Leadership: a book of readings.* Chichester: Kingsham Press; 2005.

35. Edmonstone J, Flanagan H. A flexible friend: action learning in the context of a multi-agency organisation development programme. *Action Learn Res Pract.* 2007; **4**(2): 199–209.

36. Edmonstone J. Action learning as a developmental practice for clinical leadership. *Int J Clin Leader.* 2008; **16**(2): 59–64.

37. Brook C. The role of the NHS in the development of Revans' action learning: correspondence and contradiction in action learning development and practice. *Action Learn Res Pract.* 2010; **7**(2): 181–92.

38. Scowcroft A. The problem with dissecting a frog (is that when you are finished it really doesn't look like a frog anymore). In: Edmonstone J, editor. *Clinical Leadership: a book of readings.* Chichester: Kingsham Press; 2005.

39. Cunningham G, Mackenzie H. The Royal College of Nursing Clinical Leadership Programme. In: Edmonstone J, editor. *Clinical Leadership: a book of readings.* Chichester: Kingsham Press; 2005.

40. Pokora J, Phillips A, van Zwanenberg T. GP Development in the Northern Deanery. In: Edmonstone J, editor. *Clinical Leadership: a book of readings.* Chichester: Kingsham Press; 2005.

41. Dack L. Action learning: a case study in supporting clinical leadership development. In: Edmonstone J, editor. *Clinical Leadership: a book of readings.* Chichester: Kingsham Press; 2005.

42. Jacobs J. *Systems of Survival.* New York: Random House; 1992.

43. Claxton G. Education for the learning age: a socio-cultural approach to learning to learn. In: Wells G, Claxton G, editors. *Learning for Life in the Twenty-First Century.* Oxford: Blackwell; 2002.

44. McGill I, Beaty L. *Action Learning: A Practitioner's Guide.* 2nd ed. London: Kogan Page; 2001.

Part 3: Resources

SLOW-MOTION QUESTIONING EXERCISE

This is an activity to be done with a large group of people in a 'taster' or 'starter' session to give them a flavour of action learning and to emphasise the importance of thinking about and delivering powerful questions and getting feedback on those that were most helpful.

1. Working with a large group of people (around 20) who are interested in learning more about action learning, ask them to work in groups of about four or five people. Position chairs and tables so that everyone can see everyone else. Distribute blank filing cards to everyone.

2. Ask everyone in the large group to identify a 'knotty' problem – a real service issue which they currently face and on which they would value some help. This could be phrased as *'The most important problem, issue or question facing me right now'.* Get them to write down their problem on one side of the card.

3. Get a volunteer from the large group to describe and elaborate their problem a little – a few minutes is normally enough – to give the group members some background. If the volunteer expresses the problem as a 'general' issue, the facilitator may need to get them to take personal responsibility for it by asking them to rephrase it along the lines of *'How can I.......?'* The other group members turn their cards over and listen carefully to the volunteer and do not interrupt.

4. Group members don't comment at this stage. Instead they listen and then write down a powerful question on the blank side of their card that they would like to ask the volunteer and that they think might help that person to explore the particular issue with which they are concerned and to increase their understanding of the situation.

5. In turn, each member of the large group asks their question. It is important that these are really questions – not advice-giving or problem solving. The volunteer with the problem does not try to respond to these questions but instead listens and makes notes of each question, 'starring' those that make them either wince or smile.

6. When each person has asked their question, the volunteer chooses the three or four questions which had most impact on them and which they think will be most useful in finding a way forward (or which is most interesting or intriguing).

7. The volunteer then reads out the three or four questions and says why they are important, challenging or intriguing. The volunteer might like to consider:
   ➤ Which questions they found most challenging or difficult.
   ➤ Which they found most helpful.
   ➤ Those that they can answer now.
   ➤ Those that they cannot answer now.

8. This provides useful feedback to the other group members on the relevance and utility of the questions they posed. The volunteer may choose to attempt to answer them then and there – or they may not.

9. The large group should then review the range and nature of the questions posed and whether they were, for example, open or closed, and what the major themes or angles emerging from them were. This can be expanded into a general discussion on the quality of good questions.

10. Having been modelled in the large group, the process can then be repeated within the groups of four to five people, based on the problems each person originally wrote down on their filing card.

BREAK-SPACE EXERCISE

This is an exercise designed to 'jump-start' the reflection process in action learning sets. It simply involves the facilitator suggesting that set members take about 10 minutes at the start of each set meeting where all set members close their eyes, remain silent and reflect. Reflection can either be general or focused – for example, on *'What is the most important thing that has happened to you since the set last met? Why is it so important? What might you learn from it?'*

For some set members, this may seem a distraction from the business of progress-reporting on their problem or issue, but it is probably also attributable to the awkwardness of being asked to reflect.

Alternatively, when pressure and tension begins to build within a set meeting, the facilitator may suggest a period of general or focused reflection in order to relieve the stress level and provide positive reinforcement for the purpose of the set.

LISTENING IN THE CORNER EXERCISE

1. This is a possible process by which set members can address their issue or problem. It is particularly effective where there is little evidence of listening behaviour in the set and where set members have difficulty in avoiding the 'expert' role. It enables set members to practice reflecting on a situation by stepping away from it and looking at how others tackle it. It is helpful where only one or two set members are 'in the spotlight' during a day or half-day meeting. The timings quoted are indicative only.

2. The set member with the service issue or problem that they are struggling with describes it to the others. The other set members listen, do not interrupt and take notes about whatever comes to mind as they listen, in particular focusing on what might lie 'underneath' the story being told, and also on their own feelings and associations. *(15 minutes)*

3. The set members quickly rehearse their immediate thoughts and feeling. The set member with the issue stays silent while the others are speaking, but is given the opportunity, when they are finished, to return to anything he/she thinks significant (preferably without defence or correction). Questions for clarification may also be asked at this point, provided they are not leading questions designed to suggest a solution. *(15 minutes)*

4. The set member with the problem is invited to move out of the group and away from the others and sit in the corner of the room – within earshot, but out of eyeshot. They should feel free to take notes on what they see, think and feel about what happens. The other set members discuss the issue that has been 'handed-over' and the presenter's involvement in it, as if he/she were not in the room. The aim is for them to play around with it, explore what is going on and to reflect on their thoughts and feelings about the issue. *(30 minutes)*

5. The presenter rejoins the group to use the time as he/she wishes – to pick up on certain points, ask for more information, rehearse what might happen if proposals were followed through, etc. The presenter might usefully comment on:
   ➤ What aspects of the dialogue they found most interesting, thought-provoking and useful.
   ➤ What aspects they found most challenging and difficult.
   ➤ What new insights have been generated.
   ➤ What they intend to do next. *(15 minutes)*

6. The set members (including the presenter) say what they have gained from the session. *(5 minutes)*

MAKING THE BEST USE OF AIRTIME

The ideal use of individual airtime in a set meeting involves both a divergent phase and a convergent phase. In the **divergent phase** individuals think and talk expansively about the current situation, what has been learned about attempts to make things different, what might be going on and ideas and options are freely and creatively generated. In the **convergent phase** potential ways forward are sifted and appraised until a possible course of next action emerges.

The GROW model provides a useful way of structuring airtime to best effect. GROW stands for:

➤ Goal
➤ Reality
➤ Options
➤ Wrap-up

Goal and Reality form the divergent phase and Options and Wrap-up form the convergent phase.

GOAL: Here the set member will be:

➤ Clarifying with the set what they want to get out of the session.
➤ Reminding people (if necessary) of the longer-term aim of the issue they are addressing.
➤ Stating the interim aim that they are pursuing now.

REALITY: Here, with the support of the other set members, the person with the issue will be:

➤ Expanding their understanding of the situation they are working with.
➤ Being very specific about what they did since the set last met and what happened as a result.
➤ Reflecting on their experience of implementing the actions agreed at the last set meeting (and any other actions subsequently taken) and capturing what this says about the current reality.
➤ Focussing on what worked and what made the best use of people's resources.
➤ Responding to powerful questions from other set members.
➤ Trying to maintain awareness of their assumptions and the mental models that they use (see the Ladder of Inference).
➤ Abandoning or modifying assumptions where they are not helpful or predictive.
➤ Discarding irrelevant history that does not inform ways forward.

OPTIONS: Here, the set member will be:

➤ Generating options for change that make the best use of people's resources.
➤ Thinking ahead about potential obstacles.
➤ Beginning to commit to making choices about what to do next.

WRAP-UP: Here the set member will be:

➤ Committing to action.

➤ Specifying the steps to take and the timings of these steps.

➤ Identifying the resources needed to achieve the steps.

➤ Clarifying how they will know that the steps have been achieved and that the desired outcomes have come to pass – what would others notice that would be different?

ACTION LEARNING CONSTELLATIONS

The set member presenting an issue or problem describes the context, the different stakeholders involved and related the inter-relationship challenges. When this is completed, they 'place' the other set members around the room in a constellation to represent the positions that those stakeholders currently occupy at that stage of the problem. Some will be close, others far apart, etc.

In turn, these 'proxy stakeholders' describe how it feels to be so positioned. The presenting set member then moves the proxy stakeholders to the positions which the presenter feels would be most helpful in addressing the issue. Once again the proxy stakeholders say how the new positions feel.

Finally, the presenter considers the implications of these movements in the room and considers how he or she might make them 'for real' back in the work situation.

SUPPORT/CHALLENGE MAP

This is designed to help set members get the balance between support and challenge in the work of the set 'right' for them. It may also show how that balance differs for different set members.

As part of the review at the end of the set meeting, the facilitator should ask each participant to say how they felt they had been supported in the set meeting on a scale of 0 (not supported) to 10 (totally supported). Then they should also be asked to say how they felt they had been challenged in the set meeting using the same scale – 0 (not challenged) to 10 (fully challenged).

The scores can be plotted onto a Support/Challenge Map showing where individuals experienced themselves and may well stimulate discussion about the appropriate degree of support and challenge needed in future set meetings.

Once learned the approach can, of course, be used at any time in a set meeting, either formally – by asking for scores and drawing a map, or informally by set members saying, for example 'I really feel that you are challenging me with an 8, but only supporting me with a 3'.

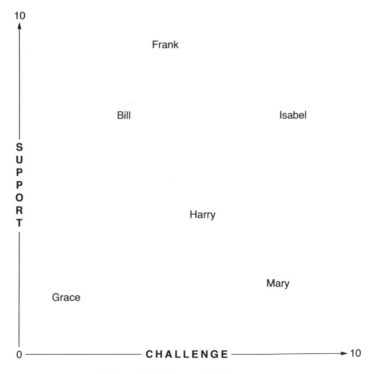

Figure 25: Support/challenge map

THINKING, FEELING AND WILLING EXERCISE

Action learning focuses on three major questions, in relation to a set member's issue or problem:

1. Who knows?
2. Who cares?
3. Who can?

These correspond with the processes of thinking, feeling and willing.

Thinking: What takes place 'in the head' – ideas, concepts, images, metaphors, theories, etc. Also, reflections, assumptions, judgements, mental models and frames of reference that lie behind the words and which cause us to see situations in particular lights.

Feeling: Emotions, sensations and energies that lie behind the words. Also, atmosphere, ambience and vibrations.

Willing: Wishes, purposes, intentions, power and energy which provides the drive, determination and effort to make things happen – the force that translates impulses and direction into practice.

The facilitator should split a large group into smaller groups of 4 people in each. One person talks for about 10–15 minutes about an issue that is important to them or about an aspect of their work they have been thinking about recently. The remaining three people listen and do not interrupt or ask questions. They simply pay attention to what the first person is saying, one each of the three concentrating on:

Thinking: What is being said by the first person, the thought-patterns – is it logical? Detailed or general? Does it refer to the past, present or future? Who is being talked about and who is not? What images and metaphors are being used? What assumptions are being made?

Feeling: What is the speaker feeling? Notice such things as gestures, posture, tone of voice, way of breathing, facial expressions and eye movement.

Willing: What does the person want to do? What is just a wish and what is a definite intention to act?

The three listeners feed-back what they each heard from the thinking, feeling and willing viewpoints to the first person, who needs to consider how what they report fits with their own perceptions.

This can then be repeated so that all four have an opportunity.

ACCESSING THE LEARNING STYLES QUESTIONNAIRE

The 80-item version of Honey & Mumfords' Learning Styles Questionnaire and the related Learning Styles Helper's Guide are available from:

Peter Honey Publications
10 Linden Avenue
MAIDENHEAD
Berkshire
SL6 6HB

Telephone: 01628-633946
Fax: 01628-633262
Email: orders@peterhoney.com
Web www.peterhoney.com

LIFE GOALS EXERCISE

This exercise is drawn from the work of Herbert Shepard on life and career planning (French & Bell, 1999).

Draw an individual 'life-line' as shown in Figure 26, where one dimension is the passage of time from the individual's birth to the present and the other relates to feelings of self-esteem, ranging from High to Low.

Prepare an inventory of important personal 'happenings', including:
➤ Any peak experiences.
➤ Things which you do well.
➤ Things which you do poorly.
➤ Things which you would like to stop doing.
➤ Things you would like to learn to do well.
➤ Peak experiences you would like to have.
➤ Values you want to live by.
➤ Things you would like to start doing now.

Take about 20 minutes to write your own obituary.

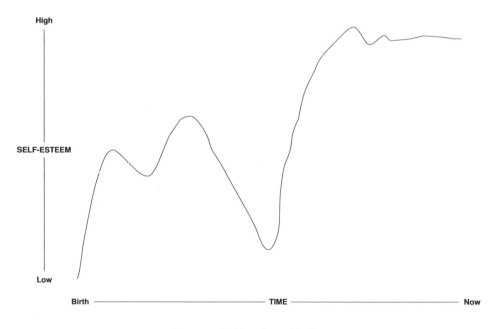

Figure 26: Drawing a life-line

CORE PROCESS EXERCISE (JONES, 1992)

➤ Divide your life into four or five sections, from birth to the present day.

➤ Recall those moments, feelings, sensations and experiences which were fulfilling and motivating – the times of feeling at one with oneself and the world.

➤ Identify the special qualities, important patterns and themes which were around at the time of these moments.

Biography approaches tend to be highly meaningful for people, who are in mid-career; who are contemplating a career or life change or who have seldom been introspective about their own lifestyle and career pattern. It should be entirely voluntary whether set members opt to undertake such work, and the caveats in Chapter 9 about means and ends also apply here.

SET MEETING REVIEW WORKSHEET

Each person should spend 5 minutes reflecting individually and privately on the work of the set at the close of the set meeting, before sharing their results with fellow set members.

My problem/issue/opportunity: The 3 key things I have learned about my problem/ issue/opportunity today are:

_____
_____
_____

Myself: The one thing I've learned about myself today is:

_____
_____
_____

Action: My action steps before the next set meeting are:

_____
_____
_____
_____
_____

Other set members: The most interesting things I have learned today about the problems/issues/opportunities facing each of the other set members are:
Name: _____
_____
_____

Name: _____
_____
_____

Name: _____
_____
_____

Name: _____
_____
_____

Name: _____
_____
_____

Name: _____
_____
_____

The set: The thing that stands out for me today in terms of the working of this set is:

_____
_____
_____

INTERNATIONAL FOUNDATION FOR ACTION LEARNING (IFAL)

The International Foundation for Action Learning was created in 1977 and is organised in chapters in the UK, USA and Canada. It offers a range of information and services related to Action Learning. The UK chapter can be contacted as follows:

Administrator
International Foundation for Action Learning
PO Box 449
ESHER
KT10 1DE

www.ifal.org.uk

ACTION LEARNING: RESEARCH AND PRACTICE

Action Learning: Research and Practice is a journal started in 2004 which seeks to publish articles which advance knowledge and assist the development of practice through action learning. It aims to address a wide audience spanning many worlds of practice. It publishes articles which aim to create theory, grounded in empirical observation of data and experience that widen the understanding of action learning in professional, community and organisational settings.

For subscription information contact:

Taylor & Francis Ltd
Customer Services Department
Rankine Road
BASINGSTOKE
Hampshire
RG24 8PR

Telephone: 01256-813002
Fax: 01256-330245
E-mail: journals.orders@tandf.co.uk
Web: www.tandf.co.uk/journals

For potential contributions please contact:

For refereed papers – Helen James

Action Learn Res Pract.
Editorial Office
Ashridge Business School
BERKHAMSTED
Hertfordshire
HP4 1NS
UK
helen.james@ashridge.org.uk

For Accounts of Practice

David Coghlan   or
FTCD School of Business
University of Dublin
Trinity College
DUBLIN 2
Ireland
dcoghlan@tcd.ie

Clare Rigg
School of Business & Social Studies
Institute of Technology
Tralee
County Kerry
Ireland
Clare.rigg@staff.ittralee.ie

The journal also acts as initiator of a bi-annual international conference on action learning run at Henley.

USEFUL WEBSITES

www.aitd.com.au/downloads/Laurie_Ormerod.pdf

www.gls.canberra.net.au/lguides/gls_lg4.pdf

www.ifal.org.uk

www.imc.org.uk

www.it.bton.ac.uk

FURTHER READING

Aspinwall K. *Evaluation Study: eighteenth month follow-up of phase 2 of the Department of Health Pathology Action Learning Programme.* Hathersage: ALSI Ltd; 2009.

Atkinson C, Landrock A. Using action learning sets to facilitate CPD in Uganda. *Occup Ther.* 2011; **19**(2): 38–40.

Attwood M. Challenging from the margins into the mainstream: improving renal services in a collaborative and entrepreneurial spirit. *Action Learn Res Pract.* 2007; **4**(2): 191–8.

Baquer A, Revans R. *But Surely that is Their Job?: a study in practical cooperation through action learning.* Southport: Action Learning Projects International Ltd; 1973.

Beattie A. Action learning for health on campus. In: Tsouros A, Dowding G, Thompson J, Dooris M, editors. *Health-Promoting Universities.* Copenhagen: World Health Organization (Europe); 1998. pp. 45–55.

Bell M, Coen E, Coyne-Nevin A, *et al.* Experiences of an action learning set. *Pract Dev Health Care.* 2007; **6**(4): 232–41.

Bering M. A personal journey into leadership. *Nurs Stand.* 2006; **13**(4): 20–5.

Billington B, Dickinson B, Durkin B, *et al. Action Learning in Hospitals for the Mentally Handicapped.* Southport: Action Learning Projects International Ltd; 1977.

Blackler F, Kennedy A. The design and evaluation of a leadership programme for experienced chief executives from the health sector. In: Rigg C, Richards S, editors. *Action Learning, Leadership and Organisational Development in Public Services.* London: Routledge; 2006.

Board M, Symons M. Community matron role development through action learning. *Primary Health Care.* 2007; **18**(8): 19–22.

Booth A, Sutton A, Falzon L. Working together: supporting projects through action learning. *Health Inform Libr J.* 2003; **20**(4): 225–31.

Boston D, Carter M. Action learning for clinical governance. *Organisations & People.* 2002; **9**(1): 22–7.

Boulden G, De Laat R. Peer group learning in Roche pharma development. *Action Learn Res Pract.* 2005; **2**(2): 197–204.

Bowerman J. Leadership development through action learning: an executive monograph. *Leader Health Serv.* 2003; **16**(4): 6–14.

Bristow N. Clinical leadership in the NHS: evaluating change through action learning. In: Hill R, Stewart J, editors. *Management Development: Perspectives from Research and Practice.* London: Routledge; 2007.

Brook C. The role of the NHS in the development of Revans' action learning: correspondence and contradiction in action learning development and practice. *Action Learn Res Pract.* 2010; **7**(2): 181–92.

Brook C. Action learning in health care. In: Dilworth R, Boshyk Y, editors. *Action Learning and Its Applications.* Basingstoke: Palgrave Macmillan; 2010.

Brook C. Action learning and change in South Manchester. *Training Journal.* 2002; **August**.

Brooks N, Moriarty A. Development of a practice learning team in the clinical setting. *Nurs Stand.* 2006; **20**(33): 41–4.

Brownlee M, Foy R. Evidence-based midwifery care: evaluation of a pilot action learning programme. *Practice Midwife.* 2000; **3**(1): 23–6.

Carlson C, Wright J. *Enabling the Development of Public Health Networks: National Public Health Network Action Learning Set Programme: summary report.* Oxford: Public Health Resource Unit, Department of Health; 2004.

Chambers N, Clark E, Smith L, *et al.* Use of action learning in a higher education setting to improve the quality of health care. *J Manag Market Healthc.* 2011; 4(1): 47–54.

Chapman A, Hosking R. *Bridging the Gap: An Action Learning Approach to Improving Care Practice.* Stirling: Dementia Services Development Centre, University of Stirling; 2009.

Charman S, McArthur M, Davies J, *et al.* '*Access for All' Action Learning Sets: evaluation report.* Bromsgrove: CAMHS Consultants/Foundation for People with Learning Disabilities; 2007.

Chivers M. Ordinary magic: developing services for children with severe communication difficulties by engaging multiple voices. *Action Learn Res Pract.* 2005; 2(1): 7–26.

Chivers M, Pedler M. *DIY Handbook for Action Learners.* Liverpool: Mersey Care NHS Trust; 2004.

Chivers M, Yates A. Towards an ecology of organisation: the impact of an action learning strategy in an NHS trust. *Paper presented at International Conference on 'Action Learning: Practices, Problems & Prospects';* Henley Management College; 2008.

Christiansen A, Robson L, Griffiths-Evans C. Creating an improvement culture for enhanced patient safety: service improvement learning in pre-registration education. *J Nurs Manag.* 2010; 18(7): 782–8.

Clark E. *Learning to Act, Learning to Listen, Listening to the Learning: using action learning to shift the balance of power within the NHS* [Unpublished PhD thesis]. Manchester: University of Manchester; 2007.

Clark E. Action learning with young carers. *Action Learn Res Pract.* 2004; 1(1): 109–16.

Clark E, Smith L, Harvey G. *Final Report of Evaluation of Action Learning for improvement in the NHS.* Coventry: NHS Institute for Innovation & Improvement; 2009.

Clarke D. *Evaluation of Practice: action learning sets for facilitators: evaluative report on the National Primary & Care Trust Transformational Change Action Learning Programme.* Salford: Revans Centre for Action Learning & Research, University of Salford for NHS Modernisation Agency; 2004.

Clarke D. *Practicing, Developing and Researching: a study of professional development through action learning* [Doctoral thesis]. Salford: Revans Institute for Action Learning & Research, University of Salford; 2002.

Clarke D, Allyson B. *Action Learning for Continuing Professional Development.* Salford: Revans Centre for Action Learning & Research, University of Salford for Institute of Healthcare Management; 2003.

Clarke D, Clarke E, Young S, *et al.* *The Selection of Action Learning Set Facilitators for Primary Care Trust Health Management.* Salford: Revans Centre for Action Learning & Research, University of Salford for NHS Modernisation Agency; 2003.

Coghill N, Stewart J. *The NHS: myth, monster or service: action learning in hospitals.* Salford: Revans Centre for Action Learning & Research, University of Salford; 1998.

Collin A, Sturt J. *Report of an Evaluation Study of an Action Learning Project in Hospitals for the Mentally Handicapped, North Derbyshire Health District.* Sheffield: Trent Regional Health Authority, Organisation Development Unit; 1978.

Cortazzi D, Baquer A. *Action Learning: a guide to its use for hospital staff.* London: King's Fund Hospital Centre; 1972.

Crofts L. Learning from experience: constructing critical case reviews for a leadership programme. *Intensive Crit Care Nurs.* 2006; **22**(5): 294–300.

Curtis-Jenkins G, White J. Action learning: a tool to improve inter-professional collaboration and promote change. *J Interprof Care.* 1994; **8**(3): 265–73.

Dack L. Action learning: a case study in supporting clinical leadership development. In: Edmonstone J, editor. *Clinical Leadership: a book of readings.* Chichester: Kingsham Press; 2005.

Davis C. Avoiding the pitfalls of action learning. *Nurse Educ Pract.* 2003; **3**(4): 183–4.

Department of Health. *Acting for Change: transforming pathology services through action learning.* London: COI; 2008.

Department of Health. *Modernising from Within: action learning solutions for pathology: learning from phase 1 of the Pathology Action Learning Programme, 2005–06.* London: Department of Health; 2007.

Department of Health. *Action Learning: transforming renal and pathology services.* London: Department of Health; 2006.

Dewing J, Wright J. A practice development project for nurses working with older people. *Pract Dev Health Care.* 2003; **2**(1): 13–28.

Donnenburg O. Network learning in an Austrian hospital. In: Pedler M, editor. *Action Learning in Practice.* 4th ed. Aldershot: Gower Publishing; 2011.

Douglas S, Machin T. A model for setting up interdisciplinary collaborative working in groups: lessons from an experience of action learning. *J Psychiatr Ment Health Nurs.* 2006; **11**: 189–93.

Down J, Hardy S. Action Learning: positive impact on patient-centred, evidence-based care and cultural change? *Paper presented at 6th International Conference on Practice Development, Action Research & Reflective Practice.* Edinburgh; 2006.

Dunphy L, Proctor G, Bartlett R, *et al.* Reflections and learning from using action learning sets in a healthcare education setting. *Action Learn Res Pract.* 2010; **7**(3): 303–14.

Du Toit S, Wilkinson A, Adam K. Role of research in occupational therapy clinical practice: applying action learning and action research in pursuit of evidence-based practice. *Aust Occ Ther J.* 2010; **57**(5): 318–30.

Edmonstone J. Action learning and organisation development. In: Pedler M, editor. *Action Learning in Practice.* 4th ed. Aldershot: Gower Publishing; 2011.

Edmonstone J. Action learning and organisation development: overlapping fields of practice. *Action Learn Res Pract.* 2011; **8**(2): 93–102.

Edmonstone J. When action learning doesn't 'take': reflections on the DALEK programme. *Action Learn Res Pract.* 2010; **7**(1): 89–97.

Edmonstone J. Action learning as a developmental practice for clinical leadership. *Int J Clin Leader.* 2008; **16**(2): 59–64.

Edmonstone J. Learning and development in action learning: the energy investment model. *Ind Commerc Train.* 2003; **35**(1): 26–8.

Edmonstone J. Problems and projects in action learning. *Ind Commerc Train.* 2002; **34**(7): 287–9.

Edmonstone J. The relevance of action learning to problem-solving and manager development in the NHS. *Health Serv Manpow Rev.* 1982; **8**(1): 16–19.

Edmonstone J, Davison V. *An Evaluation of Action Learning Sets Run for the Improvement Network, Trent Strategic Health Authority*. Ripon: MTDS; 2004.

Edmonstone J, Flanagan H. A flexible friend: action learning in the context of a multi-agency organisation development programme. *Action Learn Res Pract.* 2007; 4(2): 199–209

Edmonstone J, Mackenzie H. Practice development and action learning. *Pract Dev Health.* 2005; 4(1): 24–32.

Emerson T, Morley V, Bell C. ALS support for GP projects. *Organisations & People.* 1999; 6(3): 17–23.

Faculty of Public Health Medicine. *Learning Sets: a tool for developing a multi-agency, multi-professional approach to public health.* London: Public Health & Primary Care Group; 2001.

Faull K, Hartley L, Kalliath T. Action learning: developing a learning culture in an interdisciplinary rehabilitation team. *QE Health.* Rotorua, New Zealand; 2005.

Findlay P, Marples C. Experience in using action learning sets to enhance information management and technology strategic thinking in the UK National Health Service. *J Manag Stud.* 1998; 7(2): 165–83.

Foy R, Tidy N, Hollis S. Inter-professional learning in primary care: lessons from an action learning programme. *Br J Clin Govern.* 2002; 7(1): 40–4.

Freer J. Leadership development within an acute NHS trust. In: Edmonstone J, editor. *Clinical Leadership: a book of reading.* Chichester: Kingsham Press; 2005.

French P, Callaghan P, Dudley-Brown S, *et al.* The effectiveness of tutorials in behavioural sciences for nurses: an action learning project. *Nurs Educ Today.* 1998; 18(2): 116–24.

Giles G. Report on accreditation learning sets in the West Midlands region of the NHS. *Health Libr Rev.* 2000; 17(4): 181–8.

Graham I. Reflective practice: using the action learning group mechanism. *Nurs Educ Today.* 1995; 15(1): 28–32.

Graham I, Partlow C. Introducing and developing nurse leadership through a learning set approach. *Nurs Educ Today.* 2004; 24(6): 459–65.

Greenwood J. The role of reflection in single- and double-loop learning. *J Adv Nurs.* 1998; 27(5): 1048–53.

Griffiths W. Action learning for quality assurance – a diary: part 2. *Int J Health Care Qual Assur.* 1989; 2(1).

Griffiths W. Action learning for quality assurance – a diary: part 1. *Int J Health Care Qual Assur.* 1988; 1(3): 29–31.

Habey J. Improving patient outcomes through action learning. *Paper presented at 6th International Conference on Practice Development. Action Research & Reflective Practice.* Edinburgh; 2006.

Haddock J. Reflection in groups: contextual and theoretical considerations within nurse education and practice. *Nurs Educ Today.* 1997; 17: 381–5.

Harrison R, Miller S. The contribution of clinical directors to the strategic capability of the organisation. *Br J Manag.* 1999; 10(1): 23.

Harrison R, Miller S, Gibson A. Doctors in management – part 2: getting into action. *Exec Dev.* 1993; 6(4).

Heidari F. Action learning groups: can they help students develop their knowledge and skills? *Nurse Educ Pract.* 2003; 3(1): 49–55.

Hughes A, Elson P, Govier I. Developing practice nurses' leadership skills. *Pract Nurs.* 2006; **17**(8): 376–8.

Hunter-Jones P, Andrew P. Childhood Revisited: reflections upon the processing of information in an action learning setting. *3rd Annual Joint University of Liverpool Management School & Keele University Institute of Public Policy & Management Symposium on Current Developments in Ethnographic Research in the Social and Management Sciences.* Liverpool: University of Liverpool; 2008.

Jackson V. Medical quality management: the case for action learning as a quality initiative. *Leader Health Serv.* 2004; **17**(2): 1–8.

Jackson V. Using action learning to improve the quality of care in hospitals. *Am J Med Qual.* 2003; **18**: 104–7.

Jacobs G. 'Take control or lean back?': barriers to practising empowerment in health promotion. *Health Promotion Practitioner.* 2011; **12**(1): 94–101.

Jacobs G. The development of critical being? Reflection and reflexivity in an action learning programme for health promotion practitioners in the Netherlands. *Action Learn Res Pract.* 2008; **5**(3): 221–35.

Jenkins E, Mabbett G, Surridge A, *et al.* A co-operative inquiry into action learning and praxis development in a module for community nurses. *Qual Health Res.* 2009; **19**(9): 1303–20.

Jenkins G, White J. Action learning: a tool to improve inter-professional collaboration and promote change. *J Interprof Care.* 1994; **8**(3): 265–73.

Jones K, Bunker J, Heywood S, *et al.* Action learning to provide continuing professional development. *Nurse Prescribing.* 2005; **3**(4): 156–8.

Kellie J, Henderson E, Milsom B, *et al.* Leading change in tissue viability best practice: an action learning programme for link nurse practitioners. *Action Learn Res Pract.* 2010; **7**(2): 213–19.

Kells J. Action learning in the health and social services in Northern Ireland. *Hosp Health Serv Rev.* 1985; **81**(2): 69–71.

Kelly M, Hooke N. Help for the Helpless: the journey through action learning to becoming practice developers. *Paper presented at 6th International Conference on Practice Development. Action Research & Reflective Practice.* Edinburgh; 2006.

Kirrane C. Using action learning in reflective practice. *Prof Nurse.* 2001; **16**(5): 1102–5.

Lamont S, Brunero S, Russell R. An exploratory evaluation of an action learning set within a mental health service. *Nurse Educ Pract.* 2010; **10**(5): 298–302.

Laverty S. Helping doctors to solve problems. *BMJ Career Focus.* 2004; **329**: 59–60.

Learmonth A. Action learning as a tool for developing networks and building evidence-based practice in public health. *Action Learn Res Pract.* 2005; **2**(1): 97–104.

Learmonth A, Pedler M. Auto action learning: a tool for policy change? Building capacity across the developing regional system to improve health in the North East of England. *Health Policy.* 2004; **68**(2): 169–81.

Lee N. Action learning: a beginner's guide to the principles of action learning. *Nursing Times Learning Curve.* 1999; **3**(6): 2–3.

Lee N. Thinking reflectively: solutions through action learning. *Nurs Times.* 1999; **49**: 54–5.

Lewis R. Modernising pathology: what can action learning do for you? *Royal College of Pathologists Bulletin.* 2006; **133**: 14–16.

Lorentzon M. The NHS: myth, monster or service? Action learning in hospital. *J Nurs Manag.* 1998; **6**(5): 321.

Marlow A, Spratt C, Reilly A. Collaborative action learning: a paradoxical model for educational innovation in nursing. *Nurse Educ Pract.* 2008; **8**: 184–9.

Maslin-Prothero S, Ashby S, Rout A. *Using an Action Learning Research Approach to Evaluate and Develop Inter-professional Working Among Health and Social Care Staff, Particularly in Relation to the Care of Older People.* Keele: University of Keele; 2007.

McAndrew M. Use of an action learning model to create a dental faculty development programme. *J Dent Educ.* 2010; **74**(5): 517–23.

McAree D, Scott E. Action learning as an improved method for continuing professional development for pharmacists providing women's health care advice. *Int J Pharm Pract.* 2001; **9**: 82.

McCormack B, Henderson E, Boomer C, *et al.* Participating in a collaborative action learning (CAL) set: beginning the journey. *Action Learn Res Pract.* 2008; **5**(1): 5–19.

McCormack B, O'Connell C, Kerr C. *A Framework for Evaluating Action Learning in the Royal Hospitals Trust.* Belfast: Royal Hospitals Trust; 2003.

McKenzie C. Enhancing the care of the older person through action learning. *Paper presented at 6th International Conference on Practice Development, Action Research & Reflective Practice.* Edinburgh; 2006.

Mead M, Yearley C, Lawrence C, *et al.* Action learning: a learning and teaching method in the preparation programme for supervisors of midwives. *Action Learn Res Pract.* 2006; **3**(2): 175–86.

Moore J, Neithercut W, Mellors A, *et al.* Making the new deal for junior doctors happen. *BMJ.* 1994; **308**: 1553–5.

Nash S, Scammell J. How to use coaching and action learning to support mentors in the workplace. *Nurs Times.* 2010; **106**: 20–3.

Naylor H. *Action Learning in County Durham and Tees Valley* [Unpublished Discussion Paper]. Durham: County Durham & Tees Valley Strategic Health Authority; 2004.

Neubauer J. *Action Learning Guidebook.* London: King's Fund Management College; 1996.

Newton R, Wilkinson M. When the talking is over: using action learning. *Health Manpow Manag.* 1995; **21**(5): 34–9.

Nicolini D, Sher M, Childerstone S, *et al.* In search of the 'structure that reflects': promoting organisational reflection in a UK Health Authority. *Paper presented at 5th International Conference on Organisational Learning & Knowledge.* Lancaster University; 2003.

O'Connell C. *First Steps Towards the Development of an Inquiry Culture in an Acute Hospital using Action Learning.* London: Florence Nightingale Foundation; 2002.

Office for Health Management. *Action Learning Guide.* Dublin: Irish Republic; 2003.

Onyett S. Leadership for change. *Ment Health Rev.* 2002; **7**(4).

Pedler M. On the right course. *Health Management.* 2006; **10**(2): 24–5.

Pedler M, Abbott C. Am I doing it right? Facilitating action learning for service improvement. *Leader Health Serv.* 2008; **21**(3): 185–99.

Pedler M, Abbott C. Lean and learning: action learning for service improvement. *Leader Health Serv.* 2006; **21**(2): 87–98.

Pedler M, Attwood M. How can action learning contribute to social capital? *Action Learn Res Pract.* 2011; **8**(1): 27–39.

Pedler M, Lewis R, Mousdale S, *et al*. Renal action learning sets: a report of progress so far. *Br J Ren Med*. 2008; **13**(3): 27–31.

Phelan D, Birchall G. Action learning groups and cultural change in hospitals.*Health Care & Informat Rev*. 2001; **5**(4).

Plack M, Driscoll M, Marquez M, *et al*. Peer-facilitated virtual action learning: reflecting on critical incidents during a paediatric clerkship. *Academic Paediatrics*. 2010; **10**(2): 146–52.

Pokora J, Phillips A, van Zwanenberg T. GP Leadership Development in the Northern Deanery. In: Edmonstone J, editor. *Clinical Leadership: a book of readings*. Chichester: Kingsham Press; 2005.

Rayners D, Chisholm H, Appleby H. Developing leadership through action learning. *Nurs Stand*. 2002; **16**(29): 37–9.

Redmond B. *Reflection in Action: developing reflective practice in health & social services*. Aldershot: Ashgate; 2004.

Revans R. *Action Learning in Hospitals: diagnosis and therapy*. Maidenhead: McGraw-Hill; 1976.

Revans R. Helping each other to help the helpless: an essay in self-organisation: part 1. *Cybernetic*. 1975; **4**: 149–55.

Revans R. Helping each other to help the helpless: an essay in self-organisation: part 2. *Cybernetic*. 1975; **4**: 205–11.

Revans R, editor. *Hospitals: Communication, Choice and Change: the Hospital Internal Communication Project seen from within*. London: Tavistock Publications; 1972.

Revans R. *Standards for Morale: cause and effect in hospitals*. Oxford: Oxford University Press; 1964.

Richardson J, Ainsworth R, Allison R, *et al*. Using an action learning set to support the nurse and allied health professional consultant role. *Action Learn Res Pract*. 2008; **5**(1): 65–77.

Rivas K, Murray S. Our shared experience of implementing action learning sets in an acute clinical nursing setting: approach taken and lessons learned. *Contemp Nurse*. 2010; **35**(2): 182–7.

Roberts C. *Leadership at all Levels: An Action Learning Approach in Healthcare* [PhD dissertation]. Benedictine University.

Rogan K. The introduction of action learning into a midwifery curriculum. *Paper presented at Bournemouth University Collaborative Conference*. Bournemouth; 2003.

Rudman J, Bennis J, Jones C. Using action learning in practice development. *Paper presented at 6th International Conference on Practice Development, Action Research & Reflective Practice*. Edinburgh; 2006.

Scammell J, Nash S. How to use coaching and action learning to support mentors in the workplace. *Nurs Times*. 2010; **106**(3): 20–3.

Scowcroft A. The problem with dissecting a frog (is that when you are finished it doesn't really look like a frog anymore). In: Edmonstone J, editor. *Clinical Leadership: a book of readings*. Chichester: Kingsham Press; 2005.

Spurrell M. Consultant learning groups in psychiatry: report on a pilot study. *Psychiatr Bull*. 2000; **24**: 390–2.

Sutton D. *Action Learning in Hospitals for the Mentally Handicapped*. Southport: Action Learning Projects International Ltd; 1977.

Thomas J, Etheridge G. Using action learning to support and develop the role of matrons. *Nurs Times.* 2004; **100**(34): 36–8.

Towell D, Barnard K. *Towards an Action Learning Programme for the Development of Senior NHS Managers.* Leeds: Nuffield Centre for Health Service Studies, University of Leeds; 1976.

Walsh L, Freshwater D. Managing practice innovations in prison health care services. *Nurs Times.* 2006; **102**(7): 32.

Walsh M. How nurses perceive barriers to research implementation. *Nurs Stand.* 1997; **11**(29): 34–9.

Walsh S, Fegan C. Action learning: facilitating real change for part-time occupational therapy students. *Action Learn Res Pract.* 2007; **4**(2): 137–52.

Weiland G. *Improving Health Care Management.* Ann Arbor: Health Administration Press; 1981.

Weiland G, Leigh H, editors. *Changing Hospitals.* London: Tavistock Publications; 1971.

West P. Blackburn with Darwen action learning set: a model for improving the interface between inpatient and community teams. *Ment Health Rev.* 2005; **10**(1): 22–5.

Wilson D, Jones H. Working with GPs and hospital consultants in developing clinical leadership in a health community. In: Edmonstone J, editor. *Clinical Leadership: a book of readings.* Chichester: Kingsham Press; 2005.

Wilson V, Ho A, Walsh R. Participatory action research and action learning: changing clinical practice in nursing handover and communication. *J Children's & Young People's Nursing.* 2007; **2**: 85–92.

Wilson V, McCormack B, Ives G. Developing healthcare practice through action learning: individual and group journeys. *Action Learn Res Pract.* 2008; **5**(1): 21–38.

Wilson V, Walsh R, Ho A. Using action research and action learning to support and facilitate a change in nursing handover. *J Clin Nurs.* 2006; **3**: 35–42.

Wright S, Dolan M. Coming down from the ivory tower. *Prof Nurse.* 1991; **October**: 38–41.

Young S, Nixon E, Hinge D, *et al.* Action learning: a tool for the development of strategic skills for nurse consultants, *J Nurs Manag.* 2010; **18**(1): 105–10.

Index